NURSING a world view

NURSING a world view

Huda Abu-Saad, Ph.D., M.N., B.S.N.

Assistant Professor, Department of Nursing in
Biological Dysfunction, University of California,
San Francisco, California

Illustrated

The C. V. Mosby Company

ST. LOUIS • TORONTO • LONDON 1979

Printed in the United States of America

The C. V. Mosby Company
11830 Westline Industrial Drive, St. Louis, Missouri 63141

Library of Congress Cataloging in Publication Data

Abu-Saad, Huda, 1949-
Nursing: a world view.

Bibliography: p.
Includes index.
1. Nursing—History. I. Title.
[DNLM: 1. History of nursing. WY11.3 A165n]
RT31.A25 610.73'09 78-25860
ISBN 0-8016-0065-0

GW/CB/B 9 8 7 6 5 4 3 2 1 02/D/218

PREFACE

This book relates the story of nursing and the development of the profession from its beginning to the present. An emphasis on the international orientation of nursing and a multicultural approach to education have promoted a recognition by nurses of the need to broaden their views of the profession by study and through travel beyond their national boundaries. The growing interest in the international health movement encourages participation by professional nurses.

These considerations have led to this book. It is intended to orient the reader to past, present, and future nursing practices worldwide. Nurses, nurse educators, student nurses, scholars within and outside nursing, and others concerned with the availability of health manpower can put the profession of nursing into perspective best by examining the phenomenon of nursing as it has evolved through history. Only through such an understanding can one appreciate the close ties that exist in the nursing profession and in nursing education throughout the world.

The various chapters of this book trace the nursing movement through history and over large parts of the globe. Special attention is given to countries that took an active role in developing nursing as a self-governing profession and to the general state of nursing in the various countries.

Part I of the book gives an overview. Part II examines the development of nursing in history. The other parts include developments in Europe, America, Asia, Africa, Australia, and New Zealand, followed by a prediction of the directions in which nursing may move. The Appendix summarizes nursing in early and present times.

The touching and often heroic history of nursing has been presented in its own context. Toward this goal references in English, French, Arabic, Spanish, Dutch, German, Italian, and Greek have been researched. Also, for a clearer picture of present nursing practices, the ministries of health in the respective countries, the World Health Organization, and the International Council of Nurses were contacted for current information.

It is hoped that this book will help the reader trace the development of modern nursing in each of several countries; compare and contrast nursing practices in several countries; identify the contributions of specific persons to the development of the profession; see how general social conditions, especially those affecting the status of women, influenced the development and growth of the profession; compare present standards of nursing education in the various countries; and identify the role of the nurse in the health care delivery system of the world.

Those countries are included that, based on the resources available, have contributed to the development of nursing. Also, only those historical events that had a direct influence on the development of nursing are discussed.

Sincere thanks and appreciation are extended to Professor Margaret K. Morgan for her patience, support, and encouragement, which made this book a reality. Acknowledgment is also due Professors Gordon D. Lawrence, Amanda S. Baker, James W. Hensel, and Pauline H. Barton for their guidance. Appreciation is extended to Esther B. Jones, medical reference librarian, and her staff for their assistance in making available through Inter-Library Loan many of the references used in this book. Special gratitude is due the members of the P.E.O. Sisterhood of the State of Florida for their interest and support, the staff of the graduate school at the University of Florida whose assistance went beyond the call of duty, and Edna B. Larrick for her unlimited patience and skill in preparing the manuscript. And finally, my love and appreciation are extended to my husband, Ernst Huijer, for his help in translating documents from different languages and for his encouragement and emotional support that made the undertaking possible.

Huda Abu-Saad

CONTENTS

INTRODUCTION

The increasing complexity of life, the specialization of knowledge, the gap between developed and developing societies, and concern over health conditions throughout the world all point to the importance of communication and understanding among people, countries, and cultures. The growth of bureaucracy and collectivization and the impact of this change on the depersonalization of human lives has also heightened the need for better communication among people. The increased need for international education is an obvious result.

Present emphasis on *international education* relates to an increasing interest in *comparative education*. International education is mainly an analysis of cross-cultural educational influences and the impact that nations have on one another. *Development education,* on the other hand, focuses on programs that describe the national educational planning within the political, economic, social, and cultural milieus of the different countries. Both terms, international education and development education, are encompassed in the term *comparative education,* contributing directly or indirectly to the analysis and interpretation of educational practices and policies in the various cultures and countries in the world.

As a result, the need for a world view of nursing grows as nurses, as well as other members of the health professions, become increasingly conscious of their international role. In addition to a good scientific and technical preparation, nurses are demanding that their education include a wider knowledge of health conditions, facilities, and systems of public health and nursing in other countries. Such a broad view helps nurses to put into perspective the various health systems and defines the stages of development of their educational institutions, leading to a better appreciation of the role of nurses in the world.

An understanding of nursing developments requires a study of the international movement that includes a variety of nursing practices and provides a basis for a worldwide cooperation and friendship among nurses.

Ironically, although nursing practices in each country seem to illustrate the past or the future of nursing practices in some other country, nurses usually find much that they can share with one another.

With such an international orientation, all aspects of nursing—length and type of training, hours of duty, living accommodations, legislation and licensure, and quality and extent of communication between nurse and physician—become more understandable when examined country by country, until the various lands appear not as separate countries but as different stages of, or approaches to, the solution of a single problem: the provision of nursing care for the world.

The word "nursing" is derived from the same Latin root as "nurture." Among ancient civilizations, nursing was never a special service but an integral part of the care given to the young, the old, the helpless, the sick, or the injured. Through the ages, nursing has been associated with assistance to people in trouble.

Lesnik and Anderson define nursing as follows:

> The performance of any service (1) rendered pursuant to a consensual agreement, (2) requiring the application of principles based upon the biologic, physical, and social sciences in the supervision of a patient involving (3) the observation of symptoms and reactions, (4) the accurate recordation of facts, (5) the fulfillment of the legal orders of a duly licensed physician concerning treatments and medications with an understanding of cause and effect, (6) the accurate application of procedures and techniques with an understanding of cause and effect, and (7) the additional safeguarding of the physical and mental care of the patient by the employment of any nonremedial means, including but not limiting the health direction and the education of the patient.[4]

This definition came about as scientific discoveries progressed, making the practice of medicine more complex and putting pressure on nurses to assume more responsibility. From this change in the concept of care of the sick has emerged the professional nurse with the rights and privileges accorded persons in other professions.

Building on the Lesnik and Anderson definition, the Board of Directors of the American Nurses' Association in 1955 formulated a definition of professional nursing:

> The practice of professional nursing means the performance for compensation of any act in the observance, care, and counsel of the ill, injured, or infirm, or in the maintenance of health or prevention of illness of others, or in the supervision and teaching of other personnel, or the administration of medications and treatments as prescribed by a physician or a dentist; requiring substantial specialized judgment and skill based on knowledge and application of the principles of biologic, physical, and social science. The foregoing shall not be deemed to include acts of diagnosis and prescription of therapeutic and corrective measures.[1]

With the introduction of the term "nurse practitioner," the definition of nursing that portrays the concepts inherent in the term focuses on the ability of the nurse to do the following:

> . . . assess the health status of individuals and families through health and medical history taking physical examination, and defining of health and developmental problems; institute and provide continuity of health care to clients (patients), work with the client to ensure understanding of and compliance with the therapeutic regimen within established protocols, and recognize when to refer the client to a physician or other health care provider; provide instruction and counseling to individuals, families, and groups in the areas of health promotion and maintenance, including involving such person in the planning for health care; and work in collaboration with other health care providers and agencies to provide, and where appropriate to coordinate, services to individuals and families.[2: xiii]

The preceding statements define nursing in the United States; they do not represent an international definition. The definition of "nurse" adopted by the International Council of Nurses (ICN) in 1975 has been used as a membership criterion for ICN and is also an internationally acceptable definition of the scope of nursing practice. The definition states the following:

> A nurse is a person who has completed a program of basic nursing education and is qualified and authorized in her/his country to practice nursing. Basic nursing education is a formally recognized program of study which provides a broad and sound foundation for the practice of nursing and for postbasic education which develops specific competency. At the first level, the educational program prepares the nurse, through study of behavioral, life and nursing sciences and clinical experience, for effective practice and direction of nursing care, and for the leadership role. The first level nurse is responsible for planning, providing, and evaluating nursing care in all settings for the promotion of health, prevention of illness, care of the sick and rehabilitation; and functions as a member of the health team. In countries with more than one level of nursing personnel, the second level program prepares the nurse, through study of nursing theory and clinical practice, to give nursing care in cooperation with and under the supervision of a first level nurse.[3]

The International Council of Nurses hopes that the international definition of "nurse" will influence in years to come not only curricula of nursing schools throughout the world but the attitude of governments and other health professional groups as well.

REFERENCES

1. ANA Board approves a definition of nursing practice, American Journal of Nursing **55:**1474, 1955.
2. Capell, P., and Case, D.: Ambulatory care manual for nurse practitioners, Philadelphia, 1976, J. B. Lippincott Co.
3. ICN adopts definition of "nurse," International Nursing Review **22**(6):184, 1975.
4. Lesnik, M., and Anderson, B.: Legal aspects of nursing, Philadelphia, 1947, J. B. Lippincott Co.

PART I

Origins of the profession

Chapter 1

EVOLUTION OF NURSING

THE PRE-CHRISTIAN ERA

In a contemporary look at the history of nursing, great gaps appear. This probably results from the tendency of historians to neglect what is usual and commonplace. Nursing, as differentiated from medicine, is not mentioned in accounts of ancient times. Undoubtedly at one time medicine and nursing were united. At all times throughout the world, nursing and medicine have been parts of an existing culture, have been shaped by it, and in turn have helped to develop it. The comparative study of nursing, like comparative studies of other aspects of those cultures, can be fascinating.

Thousands of years before the Christian era the regions of Asia were the abodes of advanced civilizations. The ancient Hindus believed that the prevention of disease was more important than the cure, and their medical works contain innumerable rules of hygiene.[3]

More details of nursing are found in the Hindu records than in any other ancient chronicles. Lesson IX of Charaka-Samhita gives this exposition: "The physician, the drugs, the nurse, and the patient constitute an aggregate of four. Of what virtues each of these should be possessed, so as to become causes for the cure of the disease should be known."[3:32] Thorough mastery of the scriptures, broad experience, cleverness, and purity were the principal qualifications of a physician. The four qualifications of the attending nurse were knowledge of the manner in which drugs should be prepared and compounded for administration, cleverness, devotion to the patient waited on, and purity. However, the patient, the nurse, and the drugs were regarded as objects in the hands of the physician to achieve a cure.[3]

King Asoka, who spread Buddhism three centuries before Christ, is said to have built institutions for the care of the sick, in which the attendants were asked to be gentle in the care of their patients, to give refreshing juice, medicine, and massage, and to keep their own bodies clean.[4]

Like the Indians, the ancient Egyptians had an extensive knowledge of the arts, sciences, and medicine. The oldest medical records discovered and deciphered thus far appear to be Egyptian. Many diseases and surgical operations known today are described and classified, and more than 700 drugs of the vegetable, mineral, and animal kingdoms are enumerated in the Ebers Papyrus encyclopedia.[3]

The position of women in ancient Egypt was supposed to be better than their position before the dawn of civilization. However, no mention of nurses or hospitals is made in medical books. It seems unlikely that a nation which brought medicine, pharmacy, and sanitation to so orderly and systematic a state should not have had a nursing class.[3]

As in Egypt, the scanty records of Mesopotamia tell nothing about nursing or the presence of hospitals during that period of history. The legal aspect of Assyrian lore was given in the code of Hammurabi, King of Babylonia, about 2000 B.C. It showed an organization of medical treatment and surgery with fixed fees and definite penalties for failure to effect cures. The Assyrian pharmacopoeia also was as embracing as that of the Egyptians.[2,7]

The Jews learned much of their hygiene from the Egyptians. Certain sanitary measures practiced by Egyptians were enforced by the Jews. The Mosaic Law gave directions concerning matters of hygiene, such as rules of diet and cleanliness and hours of work and rest. The Jews and the Arabs were pioneers in preserving and even advancing medical knowledge during the period from the fall of Rome until the revival in Europe of ancient Greek and Roman learning.[6]

Like many older countries, Greece traces its medical art back to a mythical past of divine origin. The Asklepios myth, traced to 1300 B.C., depicts the medical and nursing arts present at that time. Hippocrates recognized nature and taught that disease was not the work of spirits, demons, or deities but resulted from disobedience to natural laws.[3] He showed that the true art of the physician is to assist nature in the cure. In his teaching Hippocrates spoke of the cleanliness of the bedclothes, of using powder on moist skin, and of the cleaning of the mouth. Except for the giving of drugs, the nursing care of the patient was understood by the ancient Greeks. However, because of the silence of the records, nursing by efficient and educated women is assumed to have been almost unknown in those days.[3] (See Fig. 1.)

The Romans benefited by the discoveries of the Greeks but did not make original contributions to scientific techniques. In nursing history Rome's chief importance consists of having originated hospitals for the sick or wounded in the army. The great contribution of Rome to medicine is the hospital system.[5] Of nursing there is no record, apart from the work of mili-

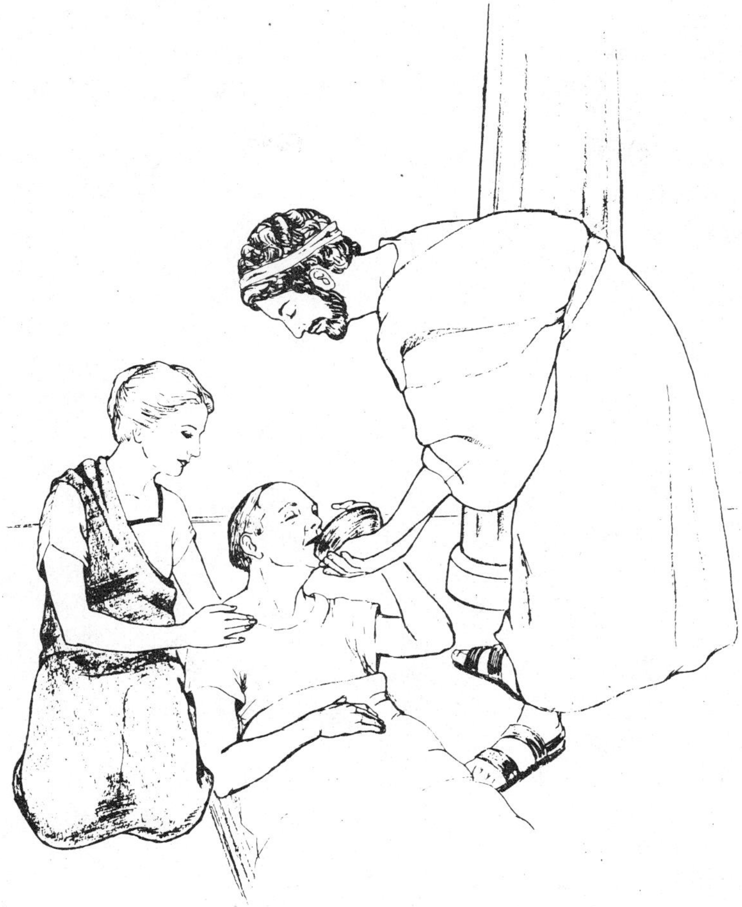

FIG. 1

Specially trained care of the sick has been a characteristic of highly civilized populations. The ancient Greeks had several centers for such care, among them the Temple of Hygeia, named for the goddess of health, the daughter of Aesculapius. (From DeLoughery, G. L.: History and trends of professional nursing, ed. 8, St. Louis, 1977, The C. V. Mosby Co.)

tary orderlies in the army. Probably in the homes of the rich, nursing was done by slaves. The diffusion of medical knowledge accumulated in the Near East, and Greece was important in the development of nursing in the Christian Era.

THE CHRISTIAN ERA

With the beginning of Christianity, the history of nursing for the first time became continuous. Christ identified the love of one's neighbor with the love of God. He stressed the care of the sick in statements such as: "I was sick and ye visited me." Illness among Christians immediately became an object of special attention. In like manner nursing was lifted to a plane of moral and religious obligation and became a respected occupation in which the most unpleasant work was ennobled by a sense of devotion to a great cause.[6]

Most active in such services were the women of the new faith. Three classifications of women were recognized as having special functions that dealt with the poor in the early church: the deaconesses, the widows, and the virgins. The deaconess carried secular as well as religious duties. Many deaconesses were women of wealth and position, probably the most famous of whom was Fabiola, who was viewed as the patron saint of early nursing. The widows, like the deaconesses, worked among the sick and the poor but apparently had less church work to perform. The virgins, on the other hand, were more concerned with church duties and religious exercises than with charitable work with the sick.[6]

The order of deaconesses of the early Christian church may well be contemplated with affectionate respect as having laid the foundations of the nurses' calling and of all modern work of charity.[3] Among women who started this calling for nursing were St. Fabiola who nursed the poor while sharing their poverty, St. Marcella who founded the first monastery for women in Rome, and St. Paula who devoted fortunes to the building of hospitals and inns for pilgrims on the way to Jerusalem. Probably no group of women ever associated with hospitals and nursing organizations has surpassed these in intellectual powers and commanding force of character.[5]

Little distinction was made in the early Christian era between caring for the sick and ministering to the poor. These activities are now shared between the professions of nursing and social work but were linked in the past, since they were seen by the church as acts of helplessness and humility requiring attention and service.[5]

Motives that led individuals into nursing were more varied than those of today. Nursing, with the dawn of Christianity, took a high place among people as a penance for sins and solace for unhappy lives.[3] However, the situation for some of the members of the group of exalted matrons whose independent positions and great wealth were used to establish community life and to organize large foundations for charity and nursing work. Roman matrons put their energies in the founding of monasteries in which women might find not only refuge and security but also a place to pursue intellectual studies or practical interests. There they could work together to establish hospitals, prepare drugs, and attend to the needs of the sick and the poor.[3]

With the rise of monasticism, medicine and nursing were taught as liberal sciences to nuns and monks who were the sole practitioners of medicine in that era. In nursing, the monks did the nursing in the men's wards and the nuns in the women's wards.[3] This arrangement prevailed all over

Western Europe, where nuns were in charge of entire hospitals. Although it cannot be claimed that much progress was made in the scientific aspects of medicine or of nursing, undoubtedly humane care administered to the sick and the needy was immensely advanced by the release of great love, the feeling of brotherhood, and the religious zeal which found expression in direct personal service to those in need. Christianity also gave women an opportunity to practice their own interests in contributing to hospital reform and charitable works.

The first religious order of men in the West was that founded by St. Benedict and known as the Benedictines. The rule of St. Benedict commanded that "before and above all things, care must be taken to the sick that they be served in very truth as Christ is served."[2:82] Benedictine monasteries spread throughout the western church and, wherever established, became of great value to local communities. These monasteries were centers of learning up to the time when universities began to develop.

In about the twelfth century a definite separation took place between establishments intended for sick persons only and those intended for the aged.[5] Many religious orders emerged as a result with the main purpose of curing the sick. These orders fell into three groups: the military nursing orders that were the outgrowth of the Crusaders, secular orders, and regular orders such as the Augustinian Sisters of the Hôtel-Dieu in Paris.[5]

As the scale of warfare in the Middle Ages increased and battles were fought in distant lands, the effects became more deadly because disease was carried wherever armies were sent. The Crusades are of special interest in this respect because they constituted the founding of the military nursing orders. The Knights of St. John, the Teutonic Knights, and the Knights of St. Lazarus were known for their contributions to military nursing and to the building of hospitals in different parts of the world.[3] The hospital service imprinted on nursing a certain military form of organization and discipline of which distinct traces are still seen.

The secular orders became active in the thirteenth century. They were not an innovation of this period, since fraternities seem to have existed and to have done nursing along with other work.[5] Orders like the Franciscans, the Carmelites, the Dominicans, and others were societies that originated outside rather than within the church. All secular orders were not devoted to nursing. However, among those which made it their main work was the Order of the Holy Ghost founded by Montpellier. This order is said to have controlled some 900 hospitals in Europe.

The Augustinian Sisters of the Hôtel-Dieu of Paris were one of the famous regular orders and one of the oldest purely nursing orders of nuns. Sisters spent their life in the wards and only went out of the hospital to do visiting nursing.[2] The literature contains little on the instructions the Sisters had for the improvement of nursing the sick and to what degree their nursing differed from domestic nursing.

THE DARK AGES OF NURSING

With the beginning of the sixteenth century, the medieval period in history ended and the modern period began. The fundamental outlook in Western Europe shifted from the God-centered, supernatural point of view to a nature-centered, or naturalistic, and secular point of view. The consequences of this change were, on the one hand, the increased material progress and invention and, on the other, a destruction of the spiritual unity of western civilization.

The confiscation of church properties by Henry the VIII of England involved the hospitals and naturally the physicians and nurses therein. The abrupt change caused by the sudden closing of hospitals during the Reformation period with the dissolution of monasteries brought with it a disorganization in the state of nursing. The wealth taken from the monastic orders was turned into institutions for the education of men. Women who were taught by nuns in convents were left out, and nurses for hospital services were drawn from the illiterate classes.[7] This reflected the temper of the time and accounted for the significant loss of interest in humane and charitable work that characterized the preceding period.

The deterioration in hospital nursing brought about by the Protestant revolt spread all over Europe. Physicians were scarce and nurses trained to help them were not available, and patients were regarded as only material for experimentation. With the coming of the Reform period, many of the humane Christian characteristics were lost. Women were subjugated and deprived of education, which was thought to be useless and disruptive to their character. Those who did nursing were middle-aged women whose time was divided among housework, laundry, scrubbing, and a pretense at nursing. Because of these and other circumstances, nursing entered a stage referred to as the "dark ages of nursing."[7:78]

This picture was relieved by the courage and farsightedness of two men, St. Vincent de Paul in 1633, a Catholic priest, and Pastor Fleidner in 1836, a Lutheran minister. In 1630 St. Vincent de Paul inaugurated a plan for instituting a society for Ladies of Charity to visit the homes and assist the sick. The members were required to be intelligent and refined young women interested in the poor and the sick; Ste. Louise de Marillac became the first director of the order. Hence, into this dark period of nursing the zeal of the Sisters of Charity became infectious and attracted many young women whose work flourished and spread, eventually encircling the globe. They performed every work of charity, including nursing in hospitals and homes, teaching in schools, taking charge of orphanages, and giving heroic service during wars.[7] (See Fig. 2.)

The Sisters of Charity were instructed in reading, writing, and arithmetic. They formed classes to discuss and question the lecture given by the physician. On graduation from the program, the Sisters were sent to other parishes as visiting nurses. St. Vincent continued counseling them not to overwork and not to take more than eight nursing cases at a time—the number modern nurses were also to find reasonable.[7]

Almost 200 years after St. Vincent established the order of the Sisters of Charity, Pastor Fleidner, influenced by the work of the deaconesses in Holland and inspired by the Sisters of Charity, established the Kaiserwerth institution. Deaconesses were prepared for many kinds of services in this order. They were taught nursing, teaching, the management of children and convalescents, including work and play activities and parish visiting and religious theory so that they could read and interpret the scriptures.[7] The Kaiserwerth deaconesses, like the Sisters of Charity, brought reform into the hospital and community nursing. Patients were treated with love and kindness and were seen as individuals, not as cases for experimentation.

Medicine, contrary to nursing, experienced considerable development during the Renaissance. The study of anatomy and physiology progressed as physicians attempted to find internal causes of disease. Obstetrics and gynecology emerged as areas of study in medical practice. Surgery, however, was regarded as inferior to medicine, resulting in a scarcity of surgeons at that time. During that period scientists emerged such as Paracel-

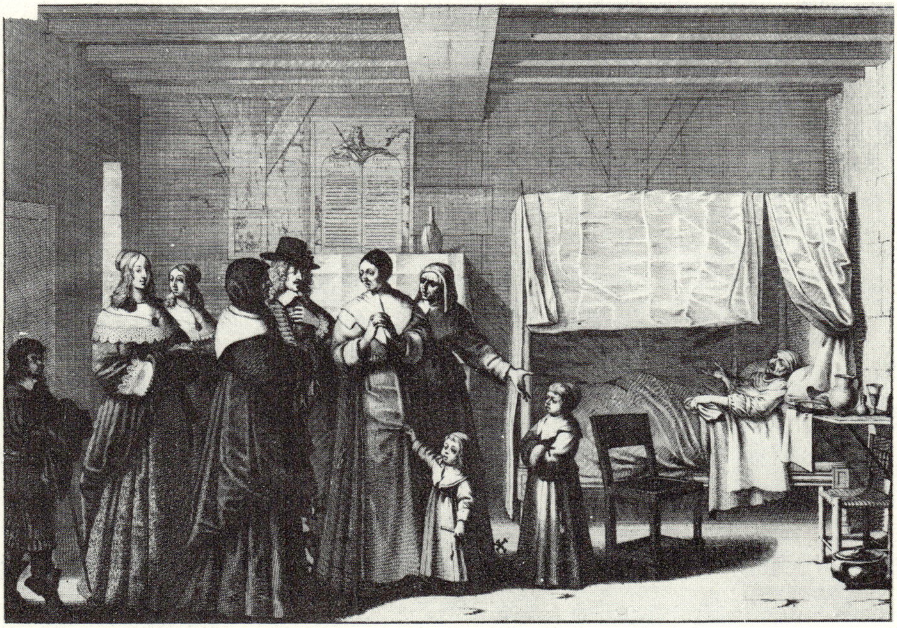

FIG. 2

Visiting the sick. (Seventeenth century copper engraving; courtesy The Bettmann Archive, Inc., New York, N.Y.)

sus, the founder of chemical pharmacology, Paré, surgeon and inventor of many surgical instruments, Vesalius, founder of the science of anatomy, and Harvey, discoverer of the circulatory system (with the exception of capillary anastomosis).[2]

The Renaissance, which revived the arts and culture, benefited medicine by renewing interest in the natural sciences. However, it hurt society by giving it a set of false values. Pleasure, leisure, and wealth were placed above work, service, and devotion. The Reformation split a united Christendom, confiscating church properties and driving out the religious and leaving the poor and the sick with no one to care for them. Although England had the worst health system at that time, it was from England that the world received a new system which improved hospitals, sanitation, and reinstated nursing.[1]

THE NIGHTINGALE REFORMS

Florence Nightingale, a leader and reformer in nursing, was born May 12, 1820, in Florence, Italy, of a well-to-do English family. She was intellectually gifted and a precocious child with a mind of her own. She was concerned from childhood with the needs of sick neighbors and members of her own family and was drawn to nursing by a strong desire to care for the sick. She wanted to establish a sort of Protestant sisterhood like the deaconess order, in which educated women would devote their lives to nursing. Her family, opposing her plan, allowed her to visit at Kaiserwerth where she was granted later a three-month training period under pastor Fleidner and his wife. There she realized her dream of practical instruction in nursing. After that training she worked for some time with the Sisters of Charity in Paris where she observed the French art of surgery.[1]

Having convinced her family of her desire to become a nurse, she took a position in charge of a private nursing home. Not long after the Crimean War broke out in 1854, Florence Nightingale was appointed superintendent of the female nursing establishment of the English General Hospital in Turkey. With the help of thirty-eight other nurses, she identified the need for change in the administration and organization of medical services of the British army. The nursing and sanitary reforms she initiated reduced the death rate from more than 400 per 1,000 patients to 22 per 1,000 patients—a rate never before known in the army even in peacetime. The soldiers loved her and felt reassured when she was nearby. Her night rounds in the hospital units gave her the title of the Lady of the Lamp. (See Fig. 3.)

Florence Nightingale's work in the Crimean War provided the basis for the modern organization of nursing and its professionalization. It brought to public attention not only the need for adequate nursing in war but the need for adequate nursing for all the sick. The fact that these needs could be met through the training of young women surprised people of the day. Florence Nightingale saw nursing as a part of a well-planned and efficiently carried out project for the health of civilians at home, men in the army, and natives of England's colonial possessions, then mainly India, Australia, New Zealand, and large areas of Africa.[7]

On her return from the Crimean War, Florence Nightingale's health did not permit her to direct in person the newly founded school of nursing. The responsibility was placed in the hands of a committee, and St. Thomas's Hospital was selected as a place to try the experiment. The new school was established amid hostile comment and criticism from the medical staff who were taking responsibility then in the training of the sisters. In spite of individual doubt and disapproval, and with the encouragement of the more enlightened members of society, the Nightingale school opened on June 15, 1860, with fifteen probationers.[7] Most significant in this respect was the recognition of science as the supreme authority in the education of a nurse.

Students of St. Thomas's received a year of training, which included instruction from the matron, the ward "sister" (head nurse), and the physicians. Next they had a two-year hospital experience, during which some probationers were paid modest salaries while gaining experience under supervision. Others, who were intended to fill higher positions later, had to

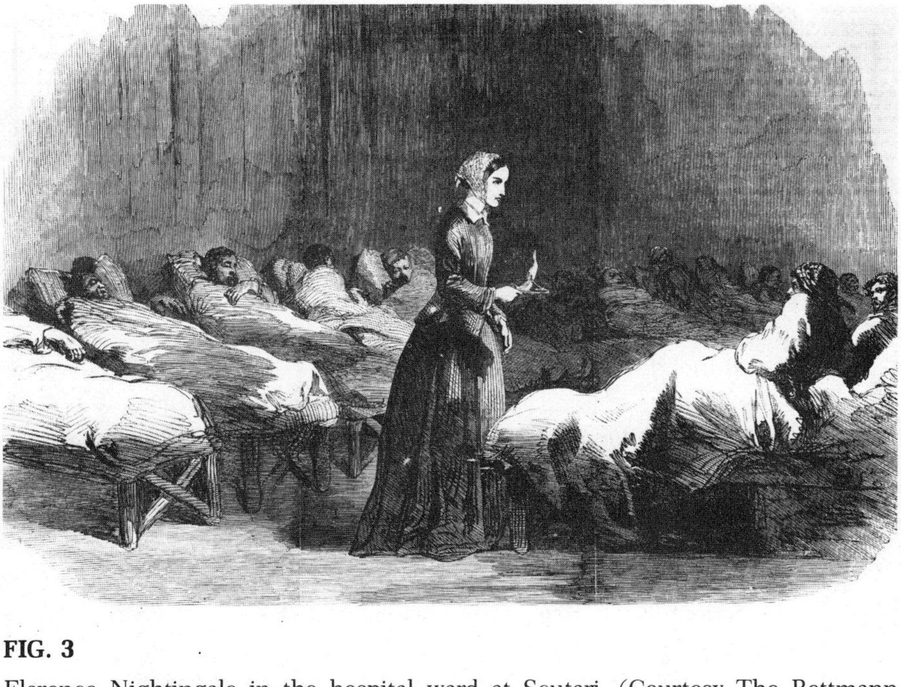

FIG. 3

Florence Nightingale in the hospital ward at Scutari. (Courtesy The Bettmann Archive, Inc., New York, N.Y.)

pay their own tuition for the first year and received a different kind of training during the following two years. The distinction between ordinary probationers and "lady nurses" reflected British class consciousness. The former group was drawn from the uneducated population, whereas the latter group were women of birth, breeding, and education. It was hoped that this system would establish public confidence in and respect for the new nurses.[7]

In administering the school of nursing, Florence Nightingale recognized two factors: the necessity of competent personnel and the adequate endowment of the school to prevent the hospital from using students for noneducational duties—two principles still strikingly important in nursing practice. The school had a Motherhouse system in which a certain degree of control was retained over the nurses after graduation. Therefore nurses were engaged through the school, which took the responsibility for the homes and institutions into which they were sent, as it did for the quality of nursing service they gave.[7]

In hospitals the Nightingale reform affected the matrons and sisters, whose responsibilities, power, and dignity were greatly enlarged. Probationers and staff nurses took the place of the old-style attendants, and ward maids, who had been doing most of the nursing, were employed for the domestic work. Night duty was started with a continuous, orderly system where graduate nurses took night shifts on an alternating basis.

Not all the movements made in nursing during that period are attributed to Florence Nightingale. Efforts in other European countries toward sanitary reform and medical progress were also noted. The Nightingale influence, however, was felt in most Protestant areas such as Holland, the Scandinavian countries, and parts of Germany. In Holland a secular nursing order started in Amsterdam in the 1880s and a Dutch Association for Sick Nursing was established in 1892.[6] On the Continent the Red Cross movement grew, as did Nightingale's movement, out of sympathy for the sufferings of sick and wounded soldiers observed by a Swiss, Jean Henri Dunant. As a result, in 1863, by the "Convention of Geneva," twelve governments founded the International Red Cross Organization. Men and women volunteers were trained to give emergency service during wars. This led later to the development of Red Cross Schools of Nursing and hospitals.[6]

In general, religious orientation continued to prevail in Catholic lands, and secular nursing orders became common in English-speaking countries. Both types of nursing flourished in Holland, Germany, and Scandinavia. Red Cross institutions, spreading at an increasing rate throughout the world, reflected whatever type of nursing existed in a given country.[6] On the whole, the standards of nursing rose throughout most parts of Europe between 1860 and 1900. Formal training became the trend, and organized lay nursing gained respectability. This trend involved extensive opportunities for women, who constituted the majority of nursing students. By the end of the nineteenth century, nursing was generally viewed as a woman's vocation.

THE NEW WORLD

European nursing standards took roots in other countries of the world. Latin America responded to French and Spanish institutions, India to the English, and Japan to general Western examples. The most conspicuous and widespread modification of the Nightingale system has been made in the United States and Canada and is referred to as the "American system." As in Britain, nursing schools in the United States were usually attached to the hospital. An exception was the role of the English matron, whose place in North America was filled by the superintendent of nurses, with responsibility for nurses in the hospital as well as the training school. Student nurses received theoretical instruction which was, on the whole, broader than that provided by the Nightingale plan.[6]

North American nursing has had no one outstanding personality such as Florence Nightingale; nevertheless, the movement fell into capable hands. The activities of three women—Lavina Dock, Isabel Hampton, and Adelaide Nutting, who founded the Nursing School at Johns Hopkins University in 1889—were remarkable at that time. From the beginning these women sought to improve theoretical instruction as well as practical training. The initiation of the *American Journal of Nursing* in 1900 by Adelaide Nutting was another important step toward a professional status. The American Nurses' Association and the National League for Nursing Education later made the periodical their official organ.[7]

Securing legal recognition for graduate nurses through registration was initiated to distinguish between graduate and nongraduate personnel. This was desirable because a large number of people—trained or untrained—were active in practicing nursing. No attempt was made by the American Nurses' Association to limit the right to practice to those who passed state examinations. As a result, standards for nursing theory and practice were set, and examining boards made up of graduate nurses were established. The title "registered nurse" (RN) was given to the graduates of authorized institutions. Educational standards improved gradually to allow the graduate nurse to secure further education, which increased the horizons of those nurses who planned to become instructors. This movement set the stage for university-level nursing outside hospital control.[7]

The accrediting of schools of nursing has been an essential means of improving programs in nursing education on all levels. The National Organization for Public Health Nursing in 1920 was the first accrediting body within the profession of nursing. In 1933 the National League for Nursing inaugurated its accrediting program.[4] The ultimate goal was to improve nursing service through the improvement of nursing education. Other specific nursing developments in the United States will be described in a separate section of this book.

REFERENCES

1. Dolan, J.: Goodnow's history of nursing, Philadelphia, 1968, W. B. Saunders Co.
2. Frank, M. C.: The historical development of nursing, Philadelphia, 1953, W. B. Saunders Co.
3. Nutting, M. A., and Dock, L. L.: A history of nursing, New York, 1910, G. P. Putnam's Sons.
4. Sellew, G., and Ebel, E.: A history of nursing, ed. 3, St. Louis, 1955, The C. V. Mosby Co.
5. Seymer, L.: A general history of nursing, London, 1935, Faber & Faber Ltd.
6. Shryock, R.: The history of nursing, Philadelphia, 1959, W. B. Saunders Co.
7. Stewart, I., and Austin, A.: A history of nursing, New York, 1962, G. P. Putnam's Sons.

ADDITIONAL READINGS

A century of nursing; reprints of four historic documents including Miss Nightingale's letter of September 18, 1872, to the Bellevue School: Foreword by Elizabeth M. Stewart and Agnes Galinas, for the National League of Nursing Education, New York, 1950, G. P. Putnam's Sons.

Cook, Sir E.: The life of Florence Nightingale, New York, 1942, The Macmillan Co.

Scovil, E. R.: Florence Nightingale's notes on nursing, American Journal of Nursing **27**:355-357, 1927.

PART II

Europe

Chapter 2

ENGLAND

Florence Nightingale's demonstration of the possibilities for nursing, followed by the success of other nurses, drew widespread attention to nursing as a profession for women that enabled the relief of suffering and service to humanity. Although British women in 1860 still suffered under some traditional handicaps and restrictions, a few broke through the taboos by finding careers in different forms of public service, most noticeably in nursing.

By 1900 the greater recognition of the value of skilled nursing had led to a greater demand for the services of nurses. In addition, the growing provision of skilled educated women ("lady nurses") to look after the poor, not only in the hospitals but also in their homes, did not go unnoticed. The urge among the upper classes to nurse the poor in the second half of the nineteenth century was accompanied by an urge to be attended by nurses when they themselves became ill.[1]

In 1859 Florence Nightingale helped William Rathbone to establish the first district nursing association in Liverpool. The three principles recommended by her and adopted by the school were as follows:

1. District nurses should have special training for their work.
2. They were not to give alms or material relief.
3. They must not interfere with the religious views of their patients.[15]

The new philanthropic movement needed time to outgrow the old concept that home visiting of the sick was a demonstration of religious charity.

In 1887 Queen Victoria's Jubilee Institute for Nurses was established to prepare nurses to work with the poor and the sick in their homes. A six-month course was offered to hospital-trained nurses on community work. Midwifery, which was considered by Florence Nightingale to be a separate vocation from nursing, created a problem to the Queen's nurses, who were confronted by maternity patients during their home visits. This led to the establishment of the Midwifery School by the Queen's Institute, which considered the trained midwives to be essential for better maternal and child care.[1]

Little attempt was made by the Nightingale school to train private nurses, and as a result, this branch of nursing never attained the same professional and social status in Britain as did hospital, district, and military nursing. In 1885, following the Public Health Act, the first industrial nurse, Phillis Flowerday, was employed by one of the factories in Britain.[15] Britain also witnessed the school nursing movement, which was started through the efforts of Amy Hughes in 1892. In spite of the prevalence of training schools, large numbers of untrained lay nurses and midwives still practiced nursing from experience, and few criteria were available whereby the general public could judge their competence.[6]

To remedy this situation, a group of "lady nurses," prompted by feelings of insecurity about their own status, banded together to introduce the first register of nurses. The purpose was to bring about a fair distinction between the trained and the untrained. The militant nurses wanted the register to draw a line between those who were fitted to practice as nurses and those who were not, raising the question of qualification. This issue was taken up by a central body of nurses, whose job was to decide which hospitals provided adequate training and which did not. In addition, a national examination was planned to ascertain whether each individual trainee had benefited from the course of study. Only those who passed the examination were to be admitted to the register.[12]

The militant "lady pupils" saw nursing as an apprenticeship, a period of trial, almost an initiation ritual, which tested who was fit to bear the title "nurse." With these objectives in mind, Mrs. Bedford Fenwick formed the British Nurses' Association and, with the help of her physician husband, secured a vote by the British Medical Association approving the registration of nurses by act of Parliament. This brought Florence Nightingale's fighting spirit back, since she believed that state licencing would lower the standards of nursing. She associated professionalism with trade unionisn, of which she disapproved. Her chief argument against the register and nurse registration was that character and morals were nonregistrable. Florence Nightingale's views were influential because many matrons in different hospitals showed vigorous opposition to registration.[1]

Such were the issues that lay beneath what nurses call "the thirty years' war"—a battle for status conducted against a background of snobbish, militant feminism.[1] In spite of all this, the lady nurses formed the British Nurses' Association with Ethel Fenwick as president. This was similar to a union of nurses made up of the elite of the profession. In 1893, to have means of expression, Ethel Fenwick assumed control and editorship of a small weekly paper called *The Nursing Record* and enlarged it in 1902 to become the *British Journal of Nursing*.[1] This journal rapidly became the foremost nursing journal in the world and the most complete record in existence of nursing affairs and progress in all countries.

The British Nurses' Association received a charter in 1893—the first given to professional women by a Queen. In 1894 the Matrons' Council of Great Britain was organized, which is represented currently by the Association of Hospital Matrons. This grew into a powerful association that was largely concerned with improvements in nursing education and organization.[1]

THE INTERNATIONAL COUNCIL OF NURSES

The International Council of Nurses (ICN) evolved from a suggestion by Ethel Fenwick during the meeting of the International Council of Women in 1899. This was supported by nurses in the United States, Canada, Denmark, Holland, South Africa, New Zealand, and Australia who attended the conference. The aim of the ICN was (1) to develop self-governing principles among nurses under nurse leadership, and (2) to develop a profession that would raise the ethical and social status of nurses. Through professional congresses the spirit of the ICN permeated a progressive and liberal attitude and stressed individuality and diversity among its members. As a result, fellowships were created to support nursing groups in their struggle for development.[15]

NURSING AND WORLD WAR I

World War I affected Britain tremendously. Nursing resources were drained to beyond the minimum requirements of civilian hospitals, with the army enrolling a large number of the trained nurses.[8] The Voluntary Aid Detachment (V.A.D.) grew out of an unprecedented need for nurses. This corps consisted of lay persons who received a short course of three to six months in first-aid nursing. The staffs of civilian hospitals were depleted as nurses left their positions to care for sick and wounded soldiers. Military hospitals had approximately one trained nurse to sixteen patients and voluntary hospitals had one trained nurse to nineteen patients.[8]

THE ROYAL COLLEGE OF NURSING

Not surprisingly, nurses became keenly concerned about developing an order in the nursing profession. Dame Sarah Swift, the chief matron of the British Red Cross Society, and the Honorable Arthur Stanley, Treasurer of St. Thomas's Hospital, took the initiative to organize the nursing profession. As a result of many efforts, the new College of Nursing came into existence in 1916. The objectives that formed the basis for its founding follow:

1. To promote better education and training of nurses and the advancement of nursing as a profession in all or any of its branches.

2. To promote uniformity of curriculum.
3. To recognize approved nursing schools.
4. To make and maintain a register of nurses to whom certificates of proficiency or of training and proficiency had been granted.
5. To promote bills in Parliament for any cause associated with interests of the nursing profession, protection, or recognition by the state.[1]

The fusion of the British Nurses' Associtation and the College of Nursing came about as a result of a statement made by Princess Christian that such a fusion would be of great advantage to the nursing profession and to the public at large. However, many leaders of the pioneer organization in Britain vigorously attacked the College of Nursing, and their position was supported by many influential nurses from other countries. In spite of this, nurse members in the College of Nursing increased in number, assuming more active leadership roles. Branches of nursing in other parts of England were developed, offering refresher courses that were then added to the program. *The Nursing Times* became the official organ of the College of Nursing and later became a weekly professional journal.[8]

The Royal College of Nursing, a national self-governing organization, was founded in 1916 and combined lay and professional groups. One of its first activities was to push through the nurses' Registration Act.[5] In addition to the general part of the Registry that was only open to women, sections were included for men, for children's nursing, fever nursing, mental nursing, and mental deficiency nursing. After the Registration Act was passed by the Parliament in 1919, the shortage of nurses was the main problem facing the hospitals and the public. In 1930 the medical journal *Lancet* appointed a commission to look into the situation. Discipline in the nursing school, which was unnecessarily severe, and the strict regulations, which were annoying to the public, were acknowledged as contributing to the shortage. Another difficulty was the conflict between the educational and the practical aspects of the training.[1]

The recommendation of the commission included better prospects for young women, the establishment of scholarships, and increased salaries for graduate nurses. The commission also suggested that arrangements should be made for nurses to join the superannuity and pension schemes. Limited hours of work per day and better admission standards were among the many recommendations. The commission was hopeful that with such reforms the crisis could be overcome and the supply of nurses would again be equal to the demand. Nursing conditions improved, undoubtedly, as a result of these recommendations.[14]

TRAINING OF ASSISTANT NURSES

In turning to other means of meeting the immediate shortage of nurses, the issue of bringing in "assistant nurses" arose. These nurses were unqualified women who varied greatly in age, skill, experience, and ability to care for the sick. Many were ex-student nurses who had not completed their training or had failed to pass the examinations. Admission of this group of nurses to the Roll was not by examination but through two years of training in an institution. The tide of World War II focused the public's attention on the status of the assistant nurses and their chance of existence as a separate entity in the nursing profession.[3]

WORLD WAR II

The outbreak of war in September, 1939, occurred at a critical time for the nursing profession. Civilian nursing problems were especially complicated and difficult, because of the high rate of war casualties during that period. Little distinction existed between civilian and military nursing, and hence many civilian nurses were assigned to nurse soldiers in the military hospitals. Early in the war the Ministry of Health set up a Civilian Nursing Reserve, which trained nurses not actively engaged in nursing, assistant nurses, and untrained volunteers. The reserve came into being early in 1939; however, by 1940 about 6,200 full-time members were at work in hospitals.[5]

A research committee's suggestion of a recruiting center and public relations department for nursing was implemented by King Edward's Hospital Fund for London. As a result, the Nursing Recruitment Center opened in April, 1940, and was headquartered in offices adjoining the College of Nursing.[3] Advisement to prospective students and public relations were the primary activities to attract more career interest in nursing. Speakers on nursing were sent to schools all over England, supplying leaflets, notes, pictures, and posters on nursing and nursing practices, These activities were coordinated with a great deal of press publicity.

In April, 1941, a division of nursing headed by a chief nursing officer was set up at the Ministry of Health. A salaries committee was established whose chief function was to draw up agreed-on scales of salaries and emoluments for the state registered nurses. The major change resulted in an increase of the salary scales of trained and experienced nurses. While these steps were being taken to improve the nurses' pay, progress was also made in the recognition of the assistant nurse. The fact that the Civilian Nursing Reserve had recruited assistant nurses for the war implied, in itself, some official recognition. This and other actions showed that relations between nurses and government officials were being strengthened.[15]

Nurse organizations were most active during the war. The Royal College of Nursing established a Committee on Nursing Reconstruction under the chairmanship of Lord Horder, the King's physician. Many monographs were issued that dealt with standards for nurse training, schools, registration, and the assistant nurse. The recommendation of the committee called for a strengthening of educational programs at all levels of nursing. The committee's report endorsed the assistant nurses and gave detailed recommendation on admission criteria, the control of the practice, and the licensing and inspection of institutions training them.[1]

Toward the end of 1942 additional measures were needed for the recruitment of nurses at all levels. A National Advisory Council for the Recruitment and Distribution of Nurses and Midwives was set up by the Ministry of Health, an indication that government departments regarded the profession of nursing as an entity with which cooperative plans could be made. Nursing officers were then appointed in the ministry to interview and advise the trained nurses.[1]

NATIONAL HEALTH SCHEME

Meanwhile plans were made for a National Health Service, which would certainly increase the demand for nurses. Under the chairmanship of Robert Wood, a committee was appointed in 1946 to examine questions such as "What is the proper task of a nurse?", "From what groups of the community should recruitment be made?", and "How can wastage during training be minimized?" Wastage, according to the committee's report, was attributed to hospital discipline, the attitude of senior staff, and the pressure of work. Results of the job analysis undertaken by the committee showed that nurses devoted 33% of their training hours in their first year to domestic duties, 24% in the second year, and 16% in the third year.[1] To enable nurses in training to be treated as students, not as maids, the committee suggested the employment of adequate hospital nursing and domestic staff who would relieve the nursing students of unnecessary chores. Another recommendation was that the course of training be dictated by the students' needs, that the financing of nurse training be independent of the hospital, and that students be under the direction of a school of nursing rather than a hospital.[1]

As a result, a Regional Nurse Training Board was established for each hospital region to plan and coordinate training facilities, coordinate standards for admission, and allocate students to training units. In addition, the boards established advisory centers to stimulate interest in the nursing profession and to advise potential nursing students. This system became the basis for the National Health Service scheme.[1]

Nationalization of health services was established in 1948. The community accepted full responsibility for the care of the sick, and hospitals became publicly owned. The central government became the sole provider of care. The country was divided into regions that were then subdivided into areas. Fourteen regional hospitals were delegated to provide hospital services. Boards took control of all the hospitals except the teaching hospitals. The Royal College of Nursing was apprehensive about all the reorganization and was among the few institutions that showed concern about possible changes in the health professions that might result. However, the majority of practicing physicians, surgeons, dentists, nurses, and other health personnel accepted appointments under the government. The National Health Service Act recognized two main categories of nurses—midwives and other health personnel. Private nurses were excluded and hence continued to offer home services when hospital conditions prevented the sick from seeking hospital care.[1,15]

THE NURSES' ACT

The Nurses' Act of 1949 created a reorganization of regional nurse training centers. For the first time treasury funds were made available for nursing education. Some smaller schools were combined to provide a wide range of experience. However, matrons of hospitals still carried responsibility for the practical experience of nursing students in the central government schools. Qualified nurses employed by the Ministry of Health took responsibility for inspecting and approving schools, determining standards of practice, and conducting examinations. Nurses in training benefited from the scheme because their hours and curriculum were improved and training allowances were granted. Married and part-time nurses were increasingly employed.[7]

The basic training of the Registry and the Roll remained focused in the hospitals because schools could not manage without trainees. Students, as a result, had little contact with the family in its natural setting. The policy that much sickness could be treated in the home was not reflected in the basic training of the nurses. Although improvements made in nurses' pay and hours of work contributed to reducing the opposition of parents and schoolteachers to nursing as a career, the working environment obviously needed a change to make it less restrictive and status ridden. Also, the government plan provided little postgraduate education in nursing. As was pointed out, the National Health Service was primarily designed for the good of the community and not for the good of those who would carry out its provisions.[1]

NURSING EDUCATION

In 1958, hospitals and public health agencies were grouped regionally to provide composite training units covering preventive and curative health aspects fundamental to nursing. The training of a student nurse entailed an introductory period of three months to cover the basic sciences, theory and practice of nursing, and educational visits to hospitals and agencies; nine weeks of pediatrics with practical experience in nursery schools and nurseries, children's outpatient departments, and wards; four weeks of obstetrics in antenatal and postnatal clinics and maternity wards;

four weeks of communicable diseases in clinics and dispensaries; ten weeks of medicine with outpatient and ward experience; thirteen weeks of surgery limited to wards and operating rooms; four weeks of gynecology; five weeks of public health with a survey of health visiting, school nursing, and home nursing; and eight weeks of psychiatry, including child guidance, outpatient department, and wards. The last six months comprised an internship in a chosen field.[4] This was planned with the intent of giving the student nurse a complete status in the profession.

Midwifery schools, like those of nursing, became separate from the hospital system. The specialized midwife was required to have the basic course of nursing before going into midwifery. A one-year training period was required. It included fifteen weeks on the general principles of midwifery, fifteen weeks on the district, attending patients in their home, and sixteen weeks on abnormal midwifery.[4] Health visiting and district nursing were regarded as specialty areas to follow the basic program. Thus hospital nursing was seen as a beginning for many other services instead of an end. The intention was to help students adapt hospital methods to home situations and to give them background knowledge of the services offered to the patient at home. These services ranged from teaching preventive methods to the follow-up of hospital discharges.[13,15]

PRESENT TRENDS IN NURSING EDUCATION

Experiments in nursing education were going on in the early 1960s. The Glasgow Royal Infirmary offered a two-year course in basic nursing, followed by a year of internship before registration was granted. This afforded no direct link with a university, but students in this plan were given full university student status. Results showed the difficulty in compressing theoretical content in two years. At the same time the Nightingale School of St. Thomas's offered a two-year training course to university graduates. Manchester University, during the same period, was offering a university course in nursing that emphasized public health and preventive health aspects. This four-year course included public health qualifications, which were usually taken on a postregistration basis. This course stressed the fact that nursing can be presented in depth as a university subject—a concept that by itself marked the beginning of a new movement in nursing which until then had been hospital oriented.[16]

In the 1970s, nurse training in England for the General Registry lasts three years and is of an apprenticeship nature. It is conducted by the nurse training school staff, which is usually a part of the hospital. At the end of the three-year period, a final examination consisting of written papers and practical work is administered. The nurse who passes it becomes eligible for registration and is given the title "State Registered Nurse" (SRN). The Roll, unlike the Registry, requires a two-year training period at the end of which the student becomes a "State Enrolled Nurse" (SEN).[14] Promotion of a staff nurse to a ward sister requires postbasic preparation, which is offered in various educational establishments outside hospitals. Postregistration courses in administration or teaching are also available for ward sisters who elect to enter administration or teaching. Such courses are offered at the Royal College of Nursing and the National Council of Nurses of the United Kingdom and last for one year.[15]

The impact of the National Health Service was not as great on nursing as was supposed because since 1923 nursing had a national training pattern and a common national examination controlled by the General Nursing Council. However, the National Health Service brought with it conformity with regard to salaries and conditions of service. It also provided great administrative opportunities for nurses at the ministerial and regional headquarter levels. The ten-year hospital building plan witnessed the emergence of nursing expertise in all fields. Nurses were on planning committees of all the building project, working with the medical team. The General Nursing Council, which is composed of registered nurses, has the responsibility of reporting to the Ministry of Health on matters of nursing. Thus the profession in England has the control of its destiny in its own hands.[10,11] A deeper inspection of the present professional scene provides encouragement. The Joint Board of Clinical Nursing Studies in England and Wales and the Committee for Clinical Nursing Studies in Scotland have planned courses for the development of nursing expertise in a number of clinical specialties.[17] Advanced practitioner courses link the clinical areas with institutions of higher education. In nursing education also the situation is far from being static. Innovation and experimentation have continued in many schools and colleges in Great Britain. Most students presently gain experience in community as well as hospital nursing and hence are better able to provide an integrated concept of nursing care. At the university level a number of integrated undergraduate degree/nursing programs have so far proved highly attractive to prospective nursing students.[17]

Another important link between nursing and higher education in Great Britain has been the considerable growth in research activities at the universities and other institutions of advanced education. Research has been mainly concerned with the profession itself—the role, function, status, and education of nurses.[17] Increasingly emphasis is also being placed on clinical aspects of investigation and manpower needs of the profession. Much of this research has been financed by the government departments whose officers have also recognized the significance of research in nursing and hence have appointed nursing research specialists. The usefulness of the research projects will be in the provision of information and hard data on which proper management of the nursing profession will be based in the future.[17]

NURSING SERVICES

At present in England each patient has a family physician, family nurse practitioner, midwife, and pediatric nurse practitioner who work together in the same premises. House calls and follow-up care are done by the visiting nurses, who are assisted by licensed practical nurses, nursing aides, and home helpers. Carefully trained in patient care, the nurses in Britain perform clinical procedures with skill that the physician sometimes cannot match. The midwives share prenatal and postnatal care with the physician, and during labor and birth they take care of all normal, uninstrumental procedures. Physicians are always on call to handle unexpected problems. The health visitor, whose position compares with that of the pediatric nurse practitioner in the United States, runs well-baby clinics and deals with minor clinical problems.[2,9]

Nursing availability and physicians' lowered work load have made it possible to treat at home many patients who might otherwise have been hospitalized. Also, the medical team presently puts more emphasis on the treatment of psychological problems, which are handled mostly by nurses who provide counseling and comforting aspects of the care beside the probing and investigating aspects. To make this service more accessible, the medical team has expanded to include social workers who take care of the patient's social problems and share them with the rest of the team.[9] Such a plan, which is widespread in England, permits more communication and coordination of health services. This in itself constitutes a solution to the National Health Service crisis, which for a time burdened the medical as well as the nursing profession.

REFERENCES

1. Abel-Smith, B.: A history of the nursing profession in Great Britain, New York, 1960, Springer Publishing Co., Inc.
2. Briggs, A.: Report of the committee on nursing, London, 1972, Her Majesty's Stationery Office.
3. Edwards, M.: Nursing in Britain, 1937-1943, American Journal of Nursing, **44:**125-135, 1944.
4. Fraser, F.: The nurse in Great Britain, Canadian Journal of Public Health, **40:** 292-301, 1949.
5. Goodall, F.: The British citizen and his nurse, Canadian Journal of Public Health **38:**151-154, 1947.
6. Goodnow, M.: Nursing history, ed. 9, Philadelphia; 1955, W. B. Saunders Co.
7. Henry, F.: Trends in England and Wales, International Nursing Review, **9:**31-33, Jan.-Feb., 1962.
8. Jensen, D. M.: History and trends of professional nursing, St. Louis, 1955, The C. V. Mosby Co.
9. Marsh, G. N.: Primary medical care: the cooperative solution to the volume problem, Journal of the American Medical Association **235**(1):45-48, 1976.
10. Nuttal, P.: Nursing in Britain, International Nursing Review **12:**6, Nov.-Dec., 1965.

11. Nuttal, P.: Nursing in England and Wales, Canadian Nurse **62:**32, 1966.
12. Nutting, M. A., and Dock, L. L.: A history of nursing, Vol. 2, New York, 1910, G. P. Putnam's Sons.
13. Schuman, M.: On the district in England, American Journal of Nursing **61:**99, 1961.
14. Sellew, G., and Ebel, E.: A history of nursing, ed. 3, St. Louis, 1955, The C. V. Mosby Co.
15. Stewart, I., and Austin, A.: A history of nursing, New York, 1962, G. P. Putnam's Sons.
16. Watkin, B.: Nursing in Britain: a year's review, Nursing Outlook **12:**56, 1964.
17. Wright, M. S.: Nursing: present perspectives and future prospects, Nursing Mirror **139**(18):53-56, 1974.

ADDITIONAL READINGS

Auld, M.: Modern trends in nursing, Nursing Mirror **142**(15):49-51, 54-55, 1976.

Brand, K. L.: Perils and parallels of women and nursing, Nursing Forum **14**(2): 160-174, 1975.

Emblin, R.: Degree courses in nursing. Part 1, Nursing Times **72:**141-143, Oct. 7, 1976.

Emblin, R.: Degree courses in nursing. Part 2, Nursing Times, **72:**145-146, Oct. 14, 1976.

Fresh perspective on nursing, Nursing Mirror **143**(4):50, 1976.

Howard, M. H.: Activity sampling in nursing, International Journal of Nursing Studies **13:**47-53, 1976.

Nursing in general practice in the re-organized national health service, Journal of the Royal College of General Practitioners **25:**593-595, 1975.

Roper, N.: An image of nursing for the 1970s, Nursing Times **72:**65-66, 1976.

Chapter 3

IRELAND

Irish hospitals and nursing extend back almost to prehistoric times. The part taken by Irish missionaries in establishing hospitals in Central Europe is well documented in history.[1] Nursing by religious orders in Ireland dates back to the fifth century when St. Brigid and her nuns attended the sick. Almost every convent and monastery then had its hospital and infirmary. Modern aspects of patient care have been noted in early Irish history. For example, the importance of peace of mind for patients was emphasized to the extent that persons and things that did not contribute to the welfare of the patient were excluded from the sickroom.[3]

The eighteenth century saw the beginning of modern municipal hospitals. Up-to-date wards, new operating rooms, and other modern appurtenances were included in most of the hospitals during that period. The institutions were served by untrained attendants, which provoked many complaints by physicians and other staff. Early in the nineteenth century the religious orders of Ireland resumed their hereditary work in nursing, and they have carried on with excellence and continuous progress in method and scope.[7] In 1835 St. Vincent's Hospital of Charity was established by Mary Aikenhead, founder of the Irish Sisters of Charity. The nursing institute of the order dates back to 1883, when four sisters were sent to the Hôpital de la Pitié in Paris to undergo a course of instruction in that nursing system.[7] These sisters were forerunners to many who joined the order later and devoted their lives to nursing the sick in the wards and instructing others in the practice of nursing.

Mother Catherine McAuley was founder of the Sisters of Mercy in Dublin in 1831. Sixteen nuns of this order went to Crimean hospitals, and some outlived Florence Nightingale there. The Sisters of Mercy recognized the need to educate nurses in modern professional methods. As a result, a school was opened in 1891 in connection with the North Infirmary of Cork, in which the sisters had complete charge.[11] This was the second secular school opened by Catholic sisters, the United States having established one earlier.[2]

The first impetus toward modern professional nursing came from the Institution for Training Nurses, founded in 1866 by Archbishop Trench and his wife. In the 1880s two schools for the training of lay nurses were founded in two old Dublin hospitals. One was headed by a Miss Franks at Madam Stevens Hospital and the other by Margaret Huxley at Sir Patrick Dun's Hospital. Opportunities for secular nursing developed slowly because nuns held most of the administrative positions in hospitals, and economic resources outside churches were limited.[7]

The Sisters of Charity School of Nursing opened in 1892 in St. Vincent's Hospital of Charity in Dublin, where the sisters themselves underwent training. The hospital staff was composed of the Sisters of Charity, who were trained by the school, having attended the lectures and passed the examination that qualified them to register. Nursing students were considered a part of the staff but were constantly supervised by matrons day and night. Their work consisted of serving for fixed periods in medical and surgical wards and attending regular courses of lectures on anatomy and physiology, hygiene, and medical and surgical nursing. To become eligible to receive the certificate of the institute, students had to pass examinations at the end of the four-year training period. Cooperative services were opened in 1906 for institute graduates who desired to remain associated with the hospital.[7] Other schools of nursing that were opened by the Sisters of Charity throughout Ireland included the Training School in the Children's Hospital in Dublin in 1892 and the school in the North Infirmary in Cork with Sister Angela as matron in 1895.[12]

The City of Dublin Nursing Institution, founded in 1884 with the aim of helping the City of Dublin Hospital, provided training and employment for Irish nurses. It supplied all the nursing in the hospital between 1884 and 1900. Madam Fitzgerald, who had been trained at the City of Dublin and later in London took up management of the institution. This pioneer institution expanded its influence in Ireland, and its branches covered a wide sphere of work. Staff nurses and probationers were sent to infirmaries in different parts of Ireland to organize nursing arrangements and staffing.[7]

Two district nursing centers, one Catholic and the other Protestant, affiliated with the Queen Victoria Jubilee Institute in Dublin. Nursing care for the poor and the sick was carried to the home on a nonsectarian basis. The *Queen's Nurses Magazine,* which originated in Ireland and was later adopted by the Queen's institute as its official publication, covered social and political events affecting nurses and their work in the community. One of the leaders in district nursing at that time was a nurse-midwife, Lady

Hermione Blackwood, who was known for her active work in Irish organization affairs.[12]

NURSING ORGANIZATION

The Irish Nurses' Association resulted from the wide distribution of nurse training, which gradually became more systematized and respected. The association started in 1900 with the establishment of a center where nurses could meet to discuss their professional affairs. Later, a committee was formed that elected Margaret Huxley as president of the organization. From this association the nurses of Dublin Club has sprung, which has come to be known for its struggle with Parliament to obtain registration for nurses. The atmosphere of teamwork and equality between physicians and nurses, and the support of the physicians for nursing problems, especially in nurse training, is impressive; it is a pleasing contrast to the story of similar developments in other countries.[12]

NURSING EDUCATION

The training of nurses in Ireland today is organized as an apprenticeship.[9] Most schools of nursing are attached to hospitals, and students function as part of the nursing team. Hospitals and schools are small, which on the one hand fosters maturity and responsibility but, on the other, provides limited experience and opportunities for advanced training. Many nurses leave Ireland after training, and many potential nurses seek training abroad.[9] Ireland was well known for its special emphasis on the mentally handicapped and mentally retarded—a dedication that reflects the influence of St. Vincent de Paul. As a result psychiatric nurse training has always been separate from that of general nurse training.

DOMICILIARY NURSING

After the disbandment of the Queen Victoria Jubilee Institute, which trained district nurses, Lady Dudley's Nursing Scheme for the establishment of district nurses in the poorest parts of Ireland was established in 1903.[9] Nurses from this institute still practice in Ireland and perform midwifery functions in different parts of the country.

The first professional organization for nurses, founded in 1925, was a branch of the National Council of Great Britain and Ireland, whose journal was *The Irish Trained Nurse and Hospital Review*. On separation from the mother branch, the National Council of Nurses in Ireland was formed, which became a member of the International Council of Nurses in 1947. A nurse registration law was then passed, to be administered by the Nursing Council of Ireland. The Nursing Act of 1950 brought about the annulment of the Midwives Act of 1918 and subsequently the virtual disappearance of the midwife in Ireland.[9,12]

THE BORD ALTRANAIS

Nursing in Ireland is governed by *An Bord Altranais* (Nursing Board), a statutory body established under the Nursing Acts of 1950 and 1961.[9] This body provides registration for all trained nurses. It also governs education and registration in basic nursing programs, develops postbasic educational programs, grants scholarships, and undertakes research in nursing. *An Bord Altranais* conducts a sixth-month course in district public health nursing for students seeking an advanced degree. A two-year nurse tutor course is offered by the National University of Ireland for nurses seeking teaching positions.[9]

An Bord Altranais is independent and self-supporting. It consists of twenty-three members, ten nurse representatives elected by the profession, and seven physicians. The remaining members represent various educational and local authorities.[12] Nurse training in Ireland is laid out by *An Bord Altranais,* and all training hospitals comply with its conditions. At present seventy recognized training hospitals exist, twenty-three in general nursing, twenty-four in psychiatric nursing, five for mentally handicapped training, and three for pediatric nurse training.[4,13] The period of training in all these hospitals is three years. Midwifery is considered a specialty and can be taken only after general nursing is completed.

TRENDS IN NURSING EDUCATION

Male nursing is newly evolving, with students concentrating mainly on nursing for psychiatric and mentally handicapped patients. Contrary to nursing trends in the world, Ireland trains only one grade of nurse.[10,13] The curricula are based on two state examinations—one taken at the end of the first year and the other at the end of the third year. Subjects studied include anatomy, physiology, surgery, medicine, psychology, psychiatry, social medicine, and other health-related subjects.[10,13] Basic education is usually organized by nurse tutors and clinical teachers. A clinical teacher course is offered by *An Bord Altranais,* whereas the nurse/tutor course is organized by the University of Dublin.[12] Postbasic education is still developing in Ireland. However, specialist courses are offered by hospitals and cover a variety of nursing areas. The candidate receives a certificate at the end of the course that allows for enrollment in the second nurse register.[13]

There is an increasing interest in the development of a university degree in nursing.[6] The University College of Galway has offered to establish a degree course in nursing—a suggestion that was received with mixed feelings by nurses. Since the postbasic program needs more developing, nurses believed that it would be difficult to accommodate the university graduates into the hospital system. In any case, plans that are newly formulated will be subject to the approval of the Ministry of Health. Another opportunity offered to the nursing profession in the past year is the development of a nursing fellowship, which was brought about by the Royal College of Surgeons in Ireland. Such a proposal means an emphasis on the development of research and an opportunity for professional advancement.[13] The whole structure of nursing in Ireland is going through change, and the near future will witness many new developments in the profession.

NATIONAL HEALTH SERVICES

A health service legislation similar to that of the British was passed in Northern Ireland in 1948. The main difference lies in its administration. The Northern Ireland General Health Services Board, appointed by the Minister of Health and local government, has the responsibility for general medical services.[5] In the Republic of Ireland the Fitzgerald Report in 1967 outlined the recommended hospital system. Since Irish hospitals are too many, too small, and too independent of each other, available resources are thus spread thinly. The plan for health services, as suggested by the report, entails the use of regional as well as general hospitals with a bed capacity ranging between 330 and 1,000 beds. These main hospitals provide acute services. County hospitals are changed to become community health centers, and district hospitals become district nursing homes. All the hospitals are integrated into one system with ascending affiliation to the regional teaching hospitals.[8]

The emphasis in this plan is obviously on the community health services, as distinct from the hospital services. However, the services of the health centers are interrelated and coordinated with hospital services for patient care. This change in the health care delivery system created considerable change in nursing education and service. As a result, nurses are working diligently to restructure the system by creating Central Colleges of Nursing instead of the available sixty-nine training institutions. University degree nursing will be the fruit of such endeavors.

REFERENCES

1. Chavasse, J.: Nursing in the Emerald Isle, International Nursing Review **15** (2):183, 1968.
2. Dock, L., and Stewart, I.: A short history of nursing, New York, 1938, G. P. Putnam's Sons.
3. Dolan, J.: History of nursing, ed. 12, Philadelphia, 1968, W. B. Saunders Co.
4. Elms, R. R.: Irish nursing at the crossroads, International Journal of Nursing Studies **11:**163-172, 1974.
5. Grey, M.: The nursing and midwifery services of Northern Ireland, International Journal of Nursing Studies **1:**145, 1964.
6. Leydon, I.: Development of nursing education in Ireland—training to meet the challenges of the future, International Journal of Nursing Studies **10:**95-101, 1973.
7. Nutting, M. A., and Dock, L. L.: A history of nursing, Vol. 2, New York, 1910, G. P. Putnam's Sons.

8. O'Carrol, M. F.: Restructuring the health care system—an Irish solution, World Hospital **7:**45-49, 1971.
9. Reidy, M.: The history of nursing in Ireland, International Nursing Review **18**(4):326-333, 1971.
10. Scanlan, M.: Nursing education in Ireland, International Nursing Review **16:** 153, April, 1969.
11. Sellew, G., and Ebel, E.: A history of nursing, ed. 3, St. Louis, 1955, The C. V. Mosby Co.
12. Stewart, I., and Austin, A.: A history of nursing, New York, 1962. G. P. Putnam's Sons.
13. Terney, B.: Nursing in Ireland, International Journal of Nursing Studies **11:** 111-117, 1974.

Chapter 4

GERMANY

Nursing in Germany, as in other European countries, was done chiefly under the auspices of religious groups—Protestant and Catholic. In the nineteenth century, hospitals were mainly under government control in spite of the fact that they were staffed by religious orders.[1] In 1836 Theodore Fleidner, pastor of a Protestant church at Kaiserwerth on-the-Rhine, introduced the German model school of nursing, which prepared deaconesses for teaching or nursing. This movement was carried later by deaconesses who transplanted it in different parts of the world. At the same time Catholic nursing orders were active in most parts of Germany.[6]

In 1863, National Red Cross societies were formed, and about forty Red Cross Hospitals were opened. These societies were active in training nurses in both short and long courses. The Motherhouse system, patterned after monasteries, was spread by the Kaiserwerth deaconesses and the Red Cross Hospitals. Nurses under this system remained associated with the schools, and governed by them, even after graduation. As a result, a great demand was placed on nurses by hospitals, and the nurses had little autonomy in such matters.[12]

With the outbreak of the Franco-Russian War in 1870, military hospitals overflowed with the injured. As a result of this, the Empress Victoria consulted Florence Nightingale in England, who sent Florence Lees, one of her expert nurses to give advice and help.[12] This led to the spread of nursing education on a broad community basis. The Victoria House, named after the Empress, was established in Berlin and incorporated many elements of the Motherhouse system. In this system nurses in training could apply for membership in a secular sisterhood. The German Red Cross followed much the same system later in reorganizing its training on a national basis. The Motherhouse of the Red Cross Sisters gave more freedom to its members, allowing them to join cultural and social activities and handle their own economic affairs, contrary to the system that was followed by the religious sisters who assumed control of the nurses who belonged to their sisterhood.[12]

THE GERMAN NURSES' ASSOCIATION

Because of dissatisfaction with policies of the Motherhouse, which was having difficulty in supporting its members, a group of nurses broke away from the mother organization and became known as "Free Sisters," or "Wild Sisters," of Germany.[5] These sisters banded together and chose Sister Agnes Karll as their leader. Through the effort of this group of nurses, the German Nurses' Association was organized in 1903 with Sister Agnes Karll as the first president. In 1906 the association published its first journal, *Unterm Lazarus Kreutz,* a militant organ of the organization. When the International Council of Nurses met in Berlin in 1904, the English, Irish, and American nurses assembled were graciously welcomed by Sister Agnes Karll.[9] This was the beginning of a friendship among nurses in the world that withstood the strain and stress of the two world wars.

Agnes Karll prepared the way for nursing to be accepted as a free and undenominational profession. She proved that nursing could be founded on ethical motives even without allegiance to the church. From the start she emphasized the importance of a three-year training program—a goal that was achieved fifty years later. Between 1909 and 1912 she was president of the International Council of Nurses and hence contributed much to the development of nursing as a profession.[4]

NURSING REGISTRATION

The German nurses, who had such difficulty in organizing, carried registration through in a surprisingly short time and with little opposition.[2] Legal regulation has always been in harmony with German philosophy and policies. This step resulted in disorganization and disorder among nurses, and nursing standards became notorious. Many nurses who took short courses from physicians and who had been practicing for some time, claimed a right to be included in the registry. This continued until the act was set by the Federal Council in 1905, abolishing short courses and calling for the training of nurses.[12] The German Registration Act required one year of study and hospital training, to be followed by a government examination at the end of the training period. In spite of all this, in Germany as a whole, persons who had hospital experience through practice and who passed the state examination, whether they had entered a school or not, were allowed to be registered.[9]

The German Nurses' Association under the leadership of Sister Agnes Karll did much to raise nursing standards and published many studies on the serious health conditions that afflicted nurses at that time. As a result of the association's strenuous efforts, the government intervened to improve working hours, salaries, and working conditions of nurses, which were described as being very poor.[12]

SOCIAL INSURANCE IN GERMANY

The development of nursing in Germany has to be considered, in part, in relation to the policies of Bismark, who forestalled the progress of socialism.[10] Social security for the working classes assumed major importance in his reign, resulting in the institution of the compulsory Social Insurance Act in 1883. This obliged wage earners and low-salaried employees in trades and occupations that are susceptible to high accident rates to seek membership in health insurance organizations. In 1923 various professional groups, including teachers and practicing nurses, were brought under the system.[10] Evidently Bismark's program was one of the earliest and most comprehensive of social insurance schemes to influence the medical and nursing fields. The health insurance plan in effect at present dates back to 1883.[1]

THE NATIONAL FEDERATION OF NURSES

When Hitler came into power in 1933, all nurses came to be included in the National Federation of Nurses and Attendants.[5] Since that time important changes have taken place in nursing organization, education, and practice. The federation comprised the Catholic nursing orders, the Protestant nursing orders or the deaconesses, the Red Cross nursing sisterhoods, the Professional Association of Nurses (The *Berufsorganisation der Krankenpflegerinnen*), The National Association of Pediatric Nurses, and the National Socialist Sisterhood of Nurses.[8] The National Council of Nursing, founded in 1936 and composed of two representatives from each of the national nursing organizations, exercised no power in determining the work of any of the previously mentioned organizations. However, through its journal *Die Deutsche Schwester* (The German Nurse), it demonstrated considerable influence on nursing practices.[12]

NURSING EDUCATION

The Nursing Act of 1938 put the education and practice of nursing on an entirely new basis.[8] A uniform nursing education was established for the entire Reich, and the practice of nursing was limited to licensed nurses. Applicants to schools of nursing, under the law, should be at least 18 years of age, must be graduates of a primary school, pass a physical examination, and prove that they had completed at least one year of work in a household of children or in a school. The nursing course extended over one and one-half years, after which the graduate nurse was obliged to continue to work under supervision for an additional year.[8] Nursing practice then was the cornerstone for nursing education. Theory supplemented practice and included lectures on ethics, anatomy and physiology, pathology, nutrition, public health nursing, and social insurance laws.[8] Physical education was compulsory for all students.

All public hospitals under the new law were to organize and maintain schools of nursing, with subsidies provided by the government when needed. The physician was the person responsible for directing activities of the school and for administering the theoretical part of the program. Graduate nurses took care of the clinical part of teaching student nurses.[12]

After Germany's defeat, different nursing groups withdrew into their own closed circles, and little attempt was made to reunite them. To have accomplished this would have been difficult in any case because Germany was then divided into four zones under British, French, American, and Russian control.[12] In American-occupied West Germany some followers of Sister Agnes Karll revived the German Nurses' Association, and in 1948 the German Nurses' Federation was formed, which included the Agnes Karll group and the Red Cross Society.[11] This newly founded association was admitted to the International Council of Nurses in 1949.[12]

COLLEGIATE NURSE TRAINING

In the early 1950s a modern collegiate school of nursing was opened at the University of Heidelberg. It still provides a broad and sound four-year basic nursing program on a university level as well as postgraduate programs in public health nursing and nursing education.[12] Training schools for the Red Cross nurses were conducted by Motherhouses. In payment for the professional training they receive, Red Cross nurses were obliged to stay with the organization for four years after graduation.[13] Public health nursing at the basic level was virtually unheard of in Germany. Health instruction and health care of patients were left in the hands of untrained assistant nurses. The Red Cross schools then took the lead in training assistant nurses, or nurses' aides, who provided a variety of services in the civilian and military domains.[13]

The general training of nurses in West Germany presently consists of a three-year course with a minimum of 1,200 hours of instruction. A final examination is usually conducted by the teaching staff and a state representative.[3] A training school is required by law to be associated with a hospital, which should provide adequate theoretical and practical training in internal medicine, surgery, gynecology, and psychiatry. Schools for children's nurses are associated in the same way with children's hospitals.[3] Training schools are headed by a matron, a senior sister, and a physician. Advanced training for nurses is not governed by law. Training for clinical specialties is organized by the hospitals in courses that range from two months to one year. Training for nurse aides lasts one year, with 250 hours of instruction. All schools of nursing are expected to be affiliated with hospitals and should be recognized by the state.[3] More emphasis is being placed on the recruitment of male students into the nursing profession—a trend developing in many parts of the world. This is attributed to the short life work span of a female nurse, averaging between five and six years, whereas that of the male nurse is forty to forty-five years. Nurse training at the university level is becoming more popular in Germany at the present time, and many German nurses hope it will be the trend in the future.

PRESENT EDUCATIONAL CONCERNS

Many concerns have been raised by professionals regarding the lack of continuity between theory and practice in the nursing field. Their main argument is that schools are emphasizing theory at the expense of practice. They believe that nursing is a practical field, the complexity of which can be acknowledged only in the light of practice, and that students can learn better in the actual situation where expectations can be fulfilled. They believe that psychomotor skills, daily routines, and communication and interaction with patients are better learned at the bedside than from books. To remedy the situation, the health professionals recommend that nurse instructors should be practitioners as well as administrators and principals of schools of nursing. In their view all incoming students should have a scientific background so that the time spent in learning nursing skills need not be interrupted. They also recommend that all nurses participate in continuing education programs to stay up to date with scientific methods.[7]

REFERENCES

1. Cowen, E.: The six: social services. Part 4, Nursing Mirror **134:**26-28, April 28, 1972.
2. Dock, L., and Stewart, I.: A short history of nursing, New York, 1938, G. P. Putnam's Sons.
3. Eichhorn, S.: Trends in the professional education of doctors, nurses, and other paramedical staff in the German Federal Republic, World Hospital **5:**77, 1969.
4. Fricke, A.: Agnes Karll, International Nursing Review **14:**43-44, June, 1967.
5. Goodnow, M.: Nursing history, ed. 9, Philadelphia, 1955, W. B. Saunders Co.
6. Jameison, E., Sewall, M., and Suhrie, E.: Trends in nursing history, ed. 6, Philadelphia 1966, W. B. Saunders Co.
7. Katscher, C.: Current status of nursing education, Deutsche Krankenpflegzeitschrift **29**(5):250-253, 1976.
8. Kroeger, G.: Nursing in Germany, American Journal of Nursing **39:**483-485, 1939.
9. Nutting, M. A., and Dock, L. L.: A history of nursing, Part 3, New York, 1910, G. P. Putnam's Sons.
10. Sellew, G., and Ebel, E.: A history of nursing, ed. 3, St. Louis, 1955, The C. V. Mosby Co.
11. Setzler, L.: Nursing and nursing education in Germany, American Journal of Nursing **45:**993-995, 1945.
12. Stewart, I., and Austin, A.: A history of nursing, New York, 1962, G. P. Putnam's Sons.
13. Weigand, E.: Nurses of the German Red Cross, American Journal of Nursing **49:**218-219, 1949.

Chapter 5

HOLLAND

EARLY TRAINING OF NURSES

In the Middle Ages, nursing of the sick in Holland was chiefly the task of religious corporations, especially those of Roman Catholic orders. For more than four centuries the Brothers of St. Johannes de Deo have devoted themselves to the care of their suffering fellow members.[16] The history of many nursing sisterhoods is also ancient. Protestant deaconesses took up the work of charity in 1830 and established their first home in 1843 in Utrecht. This movement was followed by the establishment of many other institutions that spread throughout the country. Some of these houses were later affiliated with the Kaiserwerth Association in Germany.[16] In addition to patient care in the institutions, the sisters devoted the rest of their time to district nursing.

In 1874 the White Cross Association of North Holland was formed through the efforts of many philanthropic groups. This brought about the first attempt in Holland to train women of good standing and education outside the Motherhouse system of the deaconesses. A committee on training nurses, set up by the association, was composed entirely of men. The first three nurses were trained in Amsterdam in 1879 and received certificates on the completion of the training course.[4] The high standards of this association produced many hospital reforms, which took effect in the Wilhelmina, a prominent hospital in Amsterdam, as early as 1890. These reforms were attributed to the work of a Miss Reynvaan who, like Florence Nightingale in England, emerged from a cultured home to improve the deplorable methods of nursing care.

The training of probationers and nurses at the Wilhelmina Hospital consisted of a three-year course covering basic anatomy and physiology, medical-surgical and fever nursing, first aid, foods, hygiene, and nursing ethics. Women of every class and denomination were accepted as probationers.[6] Students depended on the goodwill of nurses for instruction in the clinical areas or on their own capacity to acquire knowledge. As a result, the probationer was never considered as a student but, from the beginning of her training, was a part of the staff.[20]

Nursing was not focused solely on the hospital in Holland, since district nursing was carried out by religious as well as secular societies. Many private institutions for district nursing were founded on the broad principle of human solidarity, such as the Rotterdam, Amsterdam, and The Hague Societies for District Nursing, which sent out visiting nurses to different districts.[10] The Association of the White Cross and the Haarlem Nursing Associations also sent out private duty nurses. Nurses in the former group received fixed salaries, whereas those of the latter group had their own full fees.[15]

EARLY NURSING ORGANIZATIONS

The Dutch Association for Sick-Nursing *(de Nederlandsche Bond voor Ziekenverpleging),* founded in 1892, proposed to raise the level of nursing by bringing about order and uniformity in training and examinations. The Bond, as the association was called, had little influence in bringing about major reforms in the nursing profession. In 1899 the International Council of Nurses invited Miss Reynvaan and another nurse to attend its meeting in England.[19] In 1900 the *Nosokomos* (the Greek word for nurse) was formed with the cooperation of leading feminists and supporting physicians. A Mrs. Alertina, the first president of the *Nosokomos,* during her training at the Children's Hospital in Rotterdam, had realized how incomplete the nursing education system was and how enormous the need was for more solidarity among nurses. Her husband, Dr. Alertina, like Dr. Fenwick in England, championed the nurses' cause and, together with his wife, endeavored to unite nurses in one association and conducted campaigns to obtain better conditions for nurses.[16]

J. C. van Lanschot Hubrecht, attracted by the Alertinas, devoted her time to the advancement of the educational and ethical standards of nursing. *Nosokomis*, a militant publication of *Nosokomos,* was used by van Hubrecht to attack every stronghold of power related to the work of nursing. Efforts were being made then to achieve state registration—a movement strongly opposed by the boards of deaconesses and other groups of religious nursing orders. After many years of continuous struggle, the registration law was finally passed in 1921. Although its members were not satisfied with its details, they accepted it as a fair beginning,[17,18]

The *Nosokomos* gave keen attention to the conditions of nursing work. It urged the 8-hour schedule and declared that students should be treated as such. It instituted its own examination and insisted that nursing schools should come under the Ministry of Education. In addition, *Nosokomos* translated and published books and conducted courses for graduate nurses in obstetrics, pediatrics, public health, psychiatry, teaching, and administration.[3]

In 1928 the *Nosokomos* was replaced by a large and more inclusive organization of registered nurses called the National Association of Nurses of the Netherlands, which was accepted by the International Council of Nurses in the same year.[15] Only nurses with full general training were active voting members; all others were associate members. Training in schools then covered three years and three months. Preliminary courses were offered in the three-month period, and the actual training of the general sick-nurse took three years. This excluded obstetrics, psychiatric diseases, and public health nursing, which were offered as postgraduate courses. An admission examination was administered to all prospective students, and admission into the program was based on responses to the examination. The proportion of theory to practice in hours was 1 hour of theory to 11½ hours of practice.[11] Thus emphasis in nursing education was mainly on hospital training.

TRAINING PROGRAMS

Two types of nursing schools existed in Holland in the 1940s: those granting their graduates the "diploma A" in general nursing, which included medical, surgical, pediatric, tuberculosis, and communicable disease nursing, and those granting "diploma B" in mental nursing. A nurse with a diploma A could take the examination for a diploma B after a year and a half of training at a mental hospital. A diploma B nurse could become a diploma A nurse after a minimum of two years of training at a general hospital.[5] After completion of either the A or B diploma and after passing the state examination, the nurse received a state certificate that allowed her name to be entered in the register. She was then called a "State Registered Nurse," or *Verpleegster*.[5]

PUBLIC HEALTH NURSING

Much of the public health work in Holland was done by private agencies with state subsidies and supervision. The most important public health associations at present are the Green Cross, the White-Yellow Cross, and the Orange Cross. Trained nurses in these agencies give bedside care to patients in their homes and teach families the principles of disease prevention.[1,5] Public health training requires a basic nursing diploma and an additional one year of postgraduate work in maternity and district nursing.

PROFESSIONAL NURSING

Up to this point all training was done in the hospital. However, when training institutes were completely separated from the hospitals, professional orientation to nursing was developed with bedside training supplementing rather than dominating theoretical instruction.[14] At present, general training lasts for three and one-half years, with more emphasis placed on theory in psychology, sociology, physics, chemistry, bacteriology, pathology, and vocational training with related course work than on training as in the past. Clinical experience covers a variety of specialities, with two to six months of practice in each area. Hospital examinations are carried out at the end of every year.[7]

To secure better hours, salaries, and working conditions, nurses joined other unions. A consequence of this was the formation of a federation of professional and nonprofessional nurses' organization headed by a Miss Minelda, then president of the National Nurses' Association.[19] The appointment of a leading nurse to the Ministry of Public Health constituted the first step in bringing governmental reform into nursing practice and education.[8]

Changes in nursing education were introduced late in the 1960s. In 1969 a committee of health personnel met to discuss the status of the nursing profession. The consensus among members present, including government officials, was that:

1. Nursing education should be governed by the same law that regulates secondary education.
2. Students should be granted full status, as students and not as hospital employees.
3. Training should prepare professional nurses and should have continuity and sequence.
4. Basic nursing education should prepare graduates to function in all fields of health care.
5. The program should focus on development of the students' personality.[2:409]

These recommendations were adopted by the government early in the 1970s and are presently instituted in many cities in Holland. These programs are under the Ministry of Public Health, which exercises control over the standards of the schools. Students admitted to the intermediate nursing programs (M.B.O.) (Fig. 4), undergo a three-year training period comparable to the diploma program in the United States. This prepares them to carry on nursing functions in all nursing fields.[2]

Higher professional nursing education (H.B.O.) is another development in Holland. These programs, regulated by the Ministry of Education, offer a four-year course in basic nursing education, and although outside the university, they compare with undergraduate nursing programs in the United States. Many nursing educators are presently working to develop a university degree in nursing to prepare nurses for teaching positions in the different programs.[2]

FUTURE TRENDS

In the near future, most nursing labor in Holland will be done by graduates of the intermediate nursing programs, whereas the higher education graduates will concentrate mainly on staff functions. University graduates will be utilized for teaching positions at the two levels as well as in higher positions in the health care arena. Since secondary and higher education programs in nursing are presently under two different departments, the Ministry of Public Health and the Ministry of Education respectively, coordination is hard to achieve. The transfer of the secondary nursing program to the auspices of the Ministry of Education is one of the goals nurses are trying to achieve in Holland.[2]

HEALTH CARE SYSTEM

Health insurance covers most of the population in the Netherlands at present. Employed persons with limited income are cumpulsorily insured, the insurance covering the whole family. All persons 65 years of age and older are insured in the same way. Self-employed people with limited incomes can insure with the same companies, known as the sick funds, which cover approximately 70% of the population. The rest of the population takes up other insurance through commercial companies.[20]

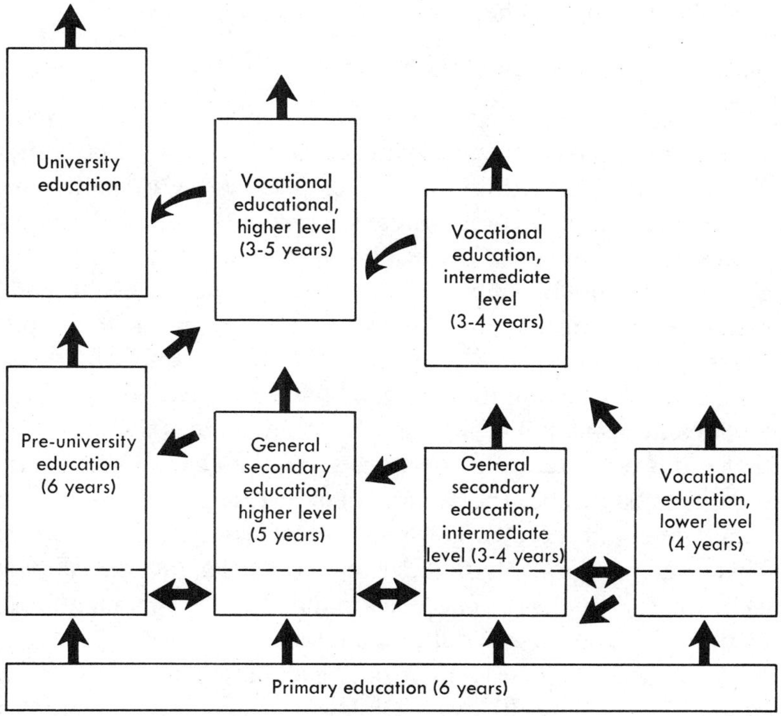

FIG. 4

Educational system in Holland. (Modified from Ministry of Education and Science, et al.: Vadmecum: a concise guide to studying in the Netherlands, The Netherlands, 1975.)

The number of nurses has increased substantially during the past twenty-five years in spite of the fact that entry requirements have become more demanding. In 1970 Holland had approximately 68,000 nurses; about 7,000 of them were men, and 750 were midwives who did approximately one third of the deliveries.[20] Graduates of the intermediate program of nursing in Holland function as family nurse practitioners and pediatric nurse practitioners. Many of these nurses work in institutions for the elderly—agencies found in abundance in the country.[2]

The central authority responsible for health services is the Ministry of Social Affairs and Public Health. Voluntary organizations with government subsidies carry on most of the preventive work in the health care delivery system. Curative care is delivered mainly by private agencies. General practitioners are private entrepreneurs, as are most of the specialists.[20] Only a minority of hospitals are presently run by the state; the majority are private, nonprofit corporations. Regionalization for the purpose of promoting coordination is emerging in Holland. This constitutes regional health care delivery systems and integration of different institutions of health care. Regionally, health care education will be the responsibility of government local officials, nursing teachers, and nursing administrators.[2]

GENERAL FRAMEWORK OF HEALTH ACTIVITIES

In Holland private agencies play a peculiar role in the delivery of preventive medicine and medical care, contrary to most countries in the world.[9] The organization of these private agencies is on a denominational basis. The Roman Catholic organizations cover one third of the population, the Protestant groups cover a little less, whereas the rest are nondenominational. The Cross organizations are the largest in public health and preventive medicine and are nationwide organizations represented by provincial officers and local branches in the municipalities. Family care as well as medical care in any field in the health profession should be provided by medical and health personnel of the same denomination as the family. This means that the Green Cross organizations serve the general group, or the nondenominational public, the White-Yellow Cross serves the Roman Catholic population, and the Orange-Green Cross serves the Protestant population. This principle in the Netherlands not only holds in medical and preventive care but also applies to hospitals founded on a denominational basis and to all fields of social and cultural life.[13]

Apart from the Cross organizations, other agencies are also involved in specific fields of health care. Child guidance clinics, marital and family guidance centers, dispensaries for alcoholics, and social and psychiatric services have infringed on the role of the nurse in the country. Nurses see to it that mental health principles are taken care of in many different kinds of health activities, such as child protection, care of unmarried mothers, care of problem families, rehabilitation of the handicapped, child health and welfare, and others. National organizations have been formed to stimulate more interest in this work. They include the Federation of Child Guidance Clinics and the Federation of Agencies for Alcohol Control, which deal with preventive mental health practice. The various national organizations that, until recently, have been functioning on a denominational basis are now preparing one joint federation to undertake all tasks in mental health care.[13]

The provincial government has the responsibility of supervising to a certain extent all the municipal agencies. Recently, provincial councils for public health have been formed and act as advisory bodies representing the local authorities. This step is intended to bring the provincial government into an active role in health matters. At the government level responsibility for public health rests with the Minister of Social Affairs and Public Health. The formulation of policy, legislation, and budgetary matters is handled by the General Directorate of Public Health.[6]

REFERENCES

1. Cowen, E. The six: social services, Nursing Mirror **134:**24-26, April 7, 1972.
2. De Haan, M. C.: The student of the intermediate professional nursing education in training and practice. 2. Nursing Education in future perspective. Tijdschrift voor Ziekenverpleging **29**(9):408-417, 1976.
3. Dock, L.: The progress of registration in Holland and Australia, American Journal of Nursing **5:**318-319, 1905.
4. Dock, L., and Stewart, I.: A short history of nursing, New York, 1938, G. P. Putnam's Sons.
5. Hooykaas, S.: Nursing in the Netherlands, American Journal of Nursing **46:** 760-762, 1946.
6. Kingdom of the Netherlands, Facts and figures, The Netherlands, 1970-1971.
7. Kruysee, M.: The training of nurses in the Wilhelmina Hospital, Amsterdam, Holland, American Journal of Nursing **2:**136-137, 1901.
8. McCarrick, H.: Holland: sense and sensibility, Nursing Times **69:**1424, 1973.
9. Meijer-Neels, E.: Part-time nursing in Holland, Nursing Mirror **106:**1149-1150, Jan. 17, 1958.
10. Melk, H. A.: A glimpse into nursing and nursing education in Holland, International Nursing Review **7:**185-188, March 8, 1932.
11. Melk, H. H.: A friendly comparison, American Journal of Nursing **30:**1103-1109, 1930.
12. Ministry of Education and Science, et al.; Vademecum: a concise guide to studying in the Netherlands, The Netherlands, 1975.
13. Ministry of Public Health and Environmental Hygiene: Mental health in the Netherlands, The Netherlands, 1972.
14. Mok, A. L.: Continuity and discontinuity in the nursing profession, International Nursing Review **16**(4):296-309, 1969.
15. Nationalen bond (pictorial), American Journal of Nursing **29:**60, 1929.
16. Nutting, M. A., and Dock. L. L.: A history of nursing, Vol. 4, New York, 1910, G. P. Putnam's Sons.

17. Sellew, G., and Ebel, E.: A history of nursing, ed. 3, St. Louis, 1955, The C. V. Mosby Co.
18. Seymer, L.: A general history of nursing, London, 1935, Faber & Faber Ltd.
19. Stewart, I., and Austin, A.: A history of nursing, New York, 1962, G. P. Putnam's Sons.
20. Stolte, E.: Health services in the Netherlands, World Hospital **6:**147, 1970.

Chapter 6

FRANCE

Throughout the early history of France, religious orders of the Catholic church did nursing among the poor and the sick. The organization of the Sisters of Charity by St. Vincent de Paul and Ste. Louise de Marillac in 1633 was an event of great significance in the history of nursing reform, growing later to become an international movement.[20] After the Franco-Prussian War in 1980, serious attempts were made in Paris by the *Assistance Publique* under a Dr. Bourneville to improve the training and practice of nursing. As a result, courses were started at the Salpêtrière and the Bicêtre in 1878 that emphasized the importance of theoretical instruction in the education of nurses. Although Dr. Bourneville did not have a woman director, such as the English matron, he was a firm believer that nursing procedures should be taught by nurses.[23] Nurse certificates were awarded at the end of the course to those who qualified by attendance and examination. Many improvements in working conditions, hours, and wages came about as a result of the continuous fight of Dr. Bourneville for reform in nursing.[24]

The establishment of the Red Cross hospitals in many European countries produced tremendous improvement in nursing practice. Nurses were trained for work in the home and for service in wartime.[20] In 1900 a small school with its paying hospital and outpatient department was established by Madam Alphen Salvador in the Rue Amyot in Paris. This school, under the *Association pour le Development de l'Assistance aux Malades,* trained young women for private duty nursing in a two-year course. A diploma was issued to students at the end of three years of hospital work.[22] In 1905 a similar Parisian school, called the Maison École d'Infirmières Privées, was started by Mademoiselle L. Chaptal. Students lived in the school where they had their lectures. Practical experience covered work done in different hospitals in the area with direct supervision from the school.[23] The *Certificat de Fin d'Etudes* was granted to the students who successfully completed the program. Both schools had a competent teaching system for the times, but the practical part of the instruction was somewhat deficient because of the lack of systematic hospital training.[7,15]

THE NIGHTINGALE SYSTEM

The Nightingale system was introduced to France in 1901 by a woman physician, Dr. Anna Hamilton. Like Florence Nightingale she was born near Florence, Italy. Her father was English; her mother was French. As a medical student, she observed crudeness and inefficiency in the care of hospital patients. Her doctoral dissertation on the care of the sick in hospitals, *Considerations sur des Infirmières Hôpitaux,* exposed the poor nursing methods and criticized the French nursing system.[9,21] Dr. Hamilton did her best to educate and enlighten public authorities on the importance of hospital training for nurses—an effort that encountered resistance by top government officials. Being a firm believer of the Nightingale system, which she had studied through visits to England, she took charge of the Maison de Santé Protestante at Bordeaux and appointed an English nurse, Catherine Elston, to head the newly organized training school, later named after Florence Nightingale.[8,11] Dr. Hamilton's plan had the full support of a Dr. Lande, mayor of the town, who was planning to establish a similar school in his municipal hospital. His school became the pioneer institution in nursing education in France.[21] Other hospitals soon followed the same program for their nurse training, which was adopted by Paris in 1907 under the direction of the Director-General of the Paris Department of Public Charities.[3]

Such a movement came about as a result of the severe conflict between Church and State, resulting in termination of the services of some religious orders that opposed the nursing reform. This was known as the *Laicisation of French Hospitals*.[3,9,24]

Dr. Hamilton's approach to the training of nurses can be summed up in the following:

1. Selection of women of education
2. Education combining lectures and ward experience that provided constant supervision of probationers
3. Simple theoretical instruction accompanying practice
4. A diploma granted upon the demonstration of theoretical as well as practical knowledge of nursing procedures
5. Designation of the trained nurse as the person responsible on the unit for carrying out staff nursing function[10:202-203]

NURSING ORGANIZATION

The social structure of France at the time was not favorable to a high and rapid development of nursing. Young French women were protected and sheltered by their parents. Thus, on the whole, they were poorly educated and tended to marry early. Recruiting educated girls for nursing was difficult; hence, candidates were obtained from the lower strata of society.[18,21] World War I broke down this convention, and as a result, more parents were willing to allow their daughters to enter the nursing profession, boosting the status of the profession considerably.[22]

The war experience in general contributed to the promotion of modern nursing in the world. Nurses of Great Britain, America, and France worked together for a common cause and exchanged ideas, which stimulated many interests for nursing improvement.[20] Mademoiselle Chaptal and Mademoiselle de Joannis, both directors of private nursing schools, became leaders of the revitalized movement. Their influence later led the French government after the war to institute a state diploma and to establish a general nursing council, which designated the requirements that schools of nursing were required to meet.[15] With the support of influential religious and civil groups, state registration became effective in 1922, giving legal recognition to nurses who had received regular training.[24] In 1923 the National Association of Graduate Nurses of France was formed, with Mademoiselle Chaptal as first president, and *L'Infirmière Française* (The French Nurse) as its official journal. In 1924 all applicants were obliged by law to pass a state examination before registration was granted.[13,22]

The association of the French nurses brought the secular and religious orders together by including nuns, protestant deaconesses, and graduates of the Nightingale, Red Cross, and other schools that offered nursing courses of two or more years' duration.[19,23] Sisters from many orders went back to training schools to take the state diploma. Four orders opened nursing schools for secular nurses and religious sisters; two were St. Vincent de Paul and the Augustinians.[15]

This group of professionals was weak compared with the large trade unions, which at the time were backed by political power. Professional nurses found it difficult to compete with the unions, especially in salaries and positions, since nonprofessional or lay nurses outnumbered trained nurses.[24] The city hospitals' nonprofessional nurses, both men and women, were grouped in a trade union affiliated with the *Confederation General du Travail*. One of their aims was the suppression of all nursing schools and the establishment of one school where anyone can join as a student nurse.[12] This went on until the French government in 1937 passed an act that forbade anyone to practice as a nurse, in a hospital or public health agency, without having the state diploma.[15]

NURSING EDUCATION

In nursing education the decree established a two-year curriculum for hospital training and three years for public health training. Schools of nursing were allowed to prepare students if they fulfilled the requirement of the adopted curriculum that stipulated practical and theoretical training, length of the training period, age of the pupils (20 to 35 years), and previous education of students with the high school diploma as the minimum level for admission. Students were to pass theoretical and practical examination before a jury of eight members chosen by the Ministry of Health.[5] At the same time the *Conseil de Perfectionnement des Écoles d'Infirmières,* (Council on Nursing Education) was formed, which studied changes and improvements to be instituted in the new curriculum. This led to curricula changes of many nursing schools that were applying to become members of the board.[5] Members of the *Conseil de Perfectionnement* were chosen from among physicians, directors of schools, public health nurses, and members of the department in the Ministry of Health responsible for health questions. In July, 1925, the Central Nursing Bureau was opened under the direction of Mademoiselle de Joannis to keep the State Register, inspect schools, and conduct examinations.[4]

In World War II, France was invaded by the Germans first, then by the Allies, resulting in the destruction of many nursing schools. When the Nazis left, many schools reopened immediately with the help of the Rockefeller Foundation and the Red Cross welfare centers.[16] In the midst of the war in 1943, France passed a law protecting the title of the registered nurse.[16,23] In 1946 another law was passed that placed the nursing profession under the Ministry of Health, giving the nurses more preference in the filling of state positions.[14]

Training of registered nurses today takes place in some 250 public or private schools, some of which are linked to hospitals. One is under the Ministry of Education; the rest are under the Ministry of Social Affairs.[1] Courses run for three years, during which nursing students receive 22 hours per week of hospital training. Theoretical instruction takes place at the school itself, usually given by physicians and nurses. Considerable emphasis in the nursing program is placed on medical and surgical pathology and on the technological aspect of nursing rather than on nursing functions that stress the psychological and comprehensive aspects of human care. On graduation most student nurses pursue paramedical studies in kinesitherapy, occupational therapy, anesthesiology, infant and child care, and social work.

POSTGRADUATE EDUCATION

The first French postgraduate school, École de Cadre pour Infirmière, was started by the French Red Cross in 1952. Such schools train nurses to become head nurses for hospital units and nursing instructors. No out-of-hospital cadre training is available.[1] In 1965 the International School for Higher Nursing Education was set up under the sponsorship of the World Health Organization. The school trains graduate nurses to assume supervisory positions in hospitals or to become directors of schools of nursing at the graduate or undergraduate levels. Training for leadership in public health nursing was also offered by the school.[1,19]

In 1967 France signed an agreement on nursing education and training, which was the result of a simultaneous action of the French National Nursing Association, the International Council of Nurses, the International Committee of Catholic Nurses and Social Workers, and the Western European Group of Nursing. The agreement allows for the reciprocal acknowledgement of nursing diplomas and for free circulation of nurses between European countries.[1] As a result of this agreement, France has witnessed what is called a "French revolution in nursing." Nursing students banded together and founded their own council in an effort to bring reforms in nursing education that included extending the period of study to three years with more emphasis on the human being rather than the almost exclusive emphasis on the ailment. This movement, which took effect in 1972, focuses on integration of courses and continuity between theory and practice.[1] Psychiatric and public health nursing, the long-forgotten fields of nursing in France, are also emerging to establish their own cadres and to claim access to basic training schools. At present the psychiatric nurse receives two years of training.[2] In France, public health nurses and social workers have always had combined jobs in what is called the *Assistante Sociale,* whose training covered the two years of study in a nursing school followed by another year and one half in a school for social workers. At present the National School of Public Health offers a one-year program to public health nurses, social workers, and midwives who have a minimum of three years' experience in their own areas of specialization.[17]

One level of nurse training is in existence at present in France with the *baccalaureat* as the acceptable level for direct entry into the program. An examination at the end of the first year is given before students are promoted to the second year. The final examination, completely under state control, is held once a year and consists of written papers in medicine and surgery, a practical examination in the hospital, and an oral test.[2] Control of the state over nurse training, examination, and registration has been complete since 1922. This is done through an advisory council on nursing affairs appointed by the Ministry of Public Health.[2]

Midwifery has been completely removed from general nursing and is regarded more as a separate profession. The training that takes place in schools of midwifery that are generally attached to medical schools, covers three years, during which examinations are given at the end of each year.[2] On completion of training, midwives can set up their own practice or obtain a position in a maternity home, which is usually run by midwives and in which most births take place.[2]

Health services have grown in much the same way throughout Western Europe. Social security, which was codified in 1945, covers the entire population. The system is presently self-supporting from contributions of employers and employees. French people can recover as much as 75% of physicians' fees, and sometimes as much as 100% is refunded if the illness is costly and lengthy.[6] The social security system retains the right of the person to choose the physician, chemist, hospital, or nurse.

REFERENCES

1. Badouaille, M. L.: Present and future position of the nursing profession in France, International Nursing Review **17**(2):146-157, 1970 (French).
2. Barrowclough, F.: The French connexion—and nursing, Nursing Times **68:** 735-736, 1972.
3. Bullough, V., and Bullough, B.: The emergence of modern nursing, ed. 2, London, 1969, The Macmillan Co.
4. Burrus, O.: The nurse in 1976; who is she? Revue de L'Infirmière **20**(4):297-304, 1976.
5. Chaptal, L.: Nursing progress in France, American Journal of Nursing **29:** 807-810, 1929.
6. Cowen, E.: The six: social services. Part 3, Nursing Mirror **134:**12-14, April 21, 1972.
7. Dock, L.: Views of nurse training and reforms in French hospitals, American Journal of Nursing **4:**61, 235-239, 1903.
8. Dock, L.: The revolution in French hospitals, American Journal of Nursing **5:**428-430, 519-522, 693-698, 887-889, 1905.
9. Dock, L.: French nurse training, American Journal of Nursing **6:**316, 1906.
10. Dock, L.: The Bordeaux School of Nursing, American Journal of Nursing **8:**202-204, 1907.
11. Dock, L.: The Florence Nightingale School in France, American Journal of Nursing **18:**1168, 1918.
12. Dock, L.: Progress in France, American Journal of Nursing **21:**393-395, 1921.
13. Dock, L.: Nursing in France, American Journal of Nursing **26:**35, 1926.
14. Dock, L.: Nursing in France, American Journal of Nursing **32:**745, 1932.
15. Dock, L., and Stewart, I.: A short history of nursing, New York, 1938, G. P. Putnam's Sons.
16. Dolan, J.: History of nursing, ed. 12, Philadelphia, 1968, W. B. Saunders Co.
17. Fautrel, F.: France: luxury and militancy, Nursing Times **69:**1345-1346, 1973.
18. Goodnow, M.: Nursing history, ed. 9, Philadelphia, 1955, W. B. Saunders Co.
19. International School for Advanced Nursing Education, Lyons, France, International Nursing Review **14:**11, Nov.-Dec., 1967.
20. Jameison, E., Sewal, M., and Suhrie, E.: Trends in nursing history, ed. 6, Philadelphia, 1966, W. B. Saunders Co.
21. Jensen, D. M.: History and trends of professional nursing, St. Louis, 1955, The C. V. Mosby Co.
22. Dellew, G., and Ebel, E.: A history of nursing, ed. 3, St. Louis, 1955, The C. V. Mosby Co.
23. Seymer, L.: A general history of nursing, London, 1935, Faber & Faber Ltd.
24. Stewart, I., and Austin, A.: A history of nursing, New York, 1962, G. P. Putnam's Sons.

Chapter 7

ITALY

Nursing in Italy, as in other European countries of the era, was done by monks and nuns. Therefore nursing was controlled by priests rather than by physicians.[2,9] Nevertheless, the servant nurses did most of the nursing care, and hospitals were staffed by cheap labor.[2] The more technical and responsible parts of nursing were done by physicians and medical students.[14] Because social restrictions surrounding young girls were more confining in Italy than in France, attempts to establish a secular nursing profession met with great resistance.

THE NIGHTINGALE INFLUENCE

The earliest Italian pioneering nursing reforms owed much to Florence Nightingale's influence. In 1895 Amy Turton, a Scottish woman and resident of Florence, corresponded with Florence Nightingale about the possibilities for reform in Italy.[6] She then spent a year as a paying probationer in the Royal Edinburgh Infirmary. On completion of her training, she decided her mission in life was to open the doors of hospitals to a new movement in secular nursing. With the help of some matrons, she succeeded in opening the first school of nursing in Rome. She then induced Grace Baxter, born in Florence of English parents and trained at Johns Hopkins Hospital in Baltimore, to open a school of nursing in Naples. Both schools started on a small scale for lay nurses. The school in Naples, later called the *Cross Azzurra* (Blue Cross), trained students who took head nurse positions in various hospitals in Italy.[3,16] A Signora Celli, a German by birth, helped the two women pioneers with her survey of Italian hospitals in which she described and criticized the nursing care in Italy. Celli wrote many articles and conducted a women's conference in which she called for nursing reform.[16]

Schools developed slowly in spite of the effort of the two pioneers. This was partly because of prejudice among the better class Italians against nursing as a profession.[5,15] However, Amy Turton did not give up. In 1910 she founded another school in Rome and put it under the direction of Dorothy Snell.[13,16] This school, later called Regina Elena, had the patronage and interest of Queen Elena and the assistance and support of the medical profession, thus becoming one of the leading schools of nursing in Italy.[19] On the whole, little reform in nursing education occurred before 1914, and all schools had difficulty developing until the social structure of Italy changed.

THE ITALIAN RED CROSS

World War I resulted in the need for lay nurses, bringing about a change of attitudes and giving Italian women freedom to choose careers. Although attempts were made in Italy before the war to organize nurses in an association, because of the scarcity of trained nurses and the disinterest of the government, efforts were fruitless. The war also initiated development of the Red Cross in Italy, and later this organization, with the help of the American Red Cross, undertook the task of promoting modern skilled nursing.[9] Mary Gardner organized public health nursing with the help of the Italian Red Cross Society. Her movement attracted into the profession many young women who hovered around the small centers she had established and tried to help in the organization as the war progressed.[12-13]

In the years that followed the war, training schools were opened by the Italian Red Cross that offered two programs in nursing. One was an internship in which students lived in the hospital where they received practical training. The other was an externship in which students stayed at home and hence received limited clinical experience. At the end of the two-year programs, students took a theoretical test that allowed them to be admitted to a postbasic degree in public health nursing.[19]

At this stage the assistance given by the Red Cross societies to the development and reforms in the nursing profession in Italy was in the following form:

1. Organizing a Corps of Voluntary Nurses, which had a strong influence in raising the prestige of nursing
2. Instituting professional schools for nurses at Milan, Rome, Bari, Bologna, Turin, and Parma
3. Putting forward legislative dispositions connected with nursing
4. Being the first to use nurses in the public health field
5. Creating nursing services with the main objective of demonstrations and experiments[18]

NURSING DECREES AND NURSING PROGRAMS

Under the Fascist regime the government became interested in nursing and moved to establish nursing standards. As a result an act was passed in 1925 that (1) recognized nursing as a profession, (2) placed nursing education under the joint responsibility of the Ministries of Interior and of

Education, (3) authorized the establishment of basic nursing schools and postgraduate courses in institutions to be approved by the two ministries, and (4) authorized the Ministry of Interior to make contributions for the functioning of these schools.[18]

In 1929 another decree was passed that regulated the governance of these schools. This was followed by a third decree in 1938 that gave the exact content the schools had to adopt in their curriculum.[18]

These government decrees resulted in the founding of the following different types of nursing programs:

1. Two-year undergraduate program leading to a professional state diploma in nursing
2. One-year postgraduate course for the training of head nurses leading to a state certificate
3. One-year postgraduate course for the training of public health nurses leading to a state diploma in public health nursing
4. Two-year course for the training of children's nurses leading to a professional diploma in children's nursing
5. Three-year course for the training of midwives leading to a professional diploma in midwifery[8,18]

NURSING ORGANIZATION AND LEGISLATION

Before the act in 1920, a group of nurses had organized a National Association for Italian Nurses, which was recognized by the Italian government at the time the act was issued. The plan then allowed nurses who met requirements of the state diploma to join the association.[6,19] In 1933 the Fascist constitution in Italy recognized state-registered nurses as belonging to a professional group rather than to a trade union. This was achieved through the strenuous efforts of the nurses' official organ *L'Infirmiara Italiana* (The Italian Nurse), coupled with the support of the physicians and professionals who believed in the advancement of nursing as a profession.[6,17]

After World War II in 1946 the Italian Nurses' Association was admitted to the International Council of Nurses as an active member with about 1,000 nurses.[6] Because of the stronghold of trade unions that supported practical and lay nurses, who were abundant at that time, a law was passed in 1954 that established a National Registration Board for Nurses, placing nursing education and practice under the Ministry of Health and Education.[7] The responsibility for the administration and supervision of nursing education was then placed in the hands of the High Commissariat. A post of nursing inspector was created in 1940 for nursing schools and services. A professional nurse was appointed to this position. Public health nurses were employed by the High Commissariat in various sections of public health service.[18]

The consequence of the Strasbourg conference in 1967 was the formulation of standard programs of nursing among the European countries. This was intended to permit free mobility of nurses among the different countries in Europe as well as the establishment of a program to meet the country's needs and, at the same time, to fall within the standards set by the conference.[11,18]

NURSING EDUCATION

The training of a nursing student at present lasts for two years and takes place in a *Convitto,* where students live. The minimum age of entry is 17 to 18 years, with secondary education as a requirement for admission.[4,10] Some nurses are paid small wages during the period of training. Lectures are mainly given by physicians and tutorial nurses, whereas clinical experience is left mainly to the nursing staff on the wards. The final state examination is given at the end of the two-year training period and consists of a written and a practical examination and an oral examination conducted by physicians. The title *Infirmiera Professionale,* which is equivalent to a State Registered Nurse, is given to students who pass.[4] In addition, a two-year course for the training of children's nurses and a three-year course for the training of midwives are also available.

One year of formal training is now available for practical nurses. Courses are organized by hospitals and conducted by physicians. Applications to these programs come mainly from domestic aides who are currently working in some hospitals in Italy. However, little difference exists between the work done by a State Registered Nurse and that done by a nonprofessional.[10]

Schools of nursing in Italy at present are like the pendulum, pulled by two main forces: the evergrowing national need for more nurses at any level of education as opposed to the long-range plans of nurse-educators for a more comprehensive program in nursing for the future. Apprehension runs high at present concerning the educational preparation of nurses, which fails to meet the country's needs. This has pointed up the importance of a sound preparation of nurse-teachers as a remedy to the perplexing problem. The organization of university programs to prepare nurse-educators is a major trend in the development of nursing in Italy. Emphasis is put on proper selection of students to such programs to have participants demonstrate proper attitudes as well as educational capabilities.[1]

REFERENCES

1. Andreoli, A.: Nursing education today, Professioni Infermieristiche **28**(4):121-124, 1976.
2. Armstrong, F. M.: The Italian hospital and nursing, American Journal of Nursing **2**:392-395, 1902.
3. Baxter, M.: A letter from Italy, American Journal of Nursing **3**:737-738, 1903.

4. Cioni, V.: Italy: Hot temper and cold baths, Nursing Times **69:**1382-1383, 1973.
5. Di Targiani-Giunti, M.: Notes on the history of nursing care with a special reference to Italy, International Nursing Review **4:**12-15, May, 1957.
6. Dock, L., and Stewart, I.: A short history of nursing, New York, 1938, G. P. Putnam's Sons.
7. Enriques, B.: Les infirmières professionelles en Italie et leur preparation, International Nursing Review **4:**15-18, May, 1957 (French).
8. Fitzgerald, A.: Congratulations to Italian nurses, American Journal of Nursing **26:**30, 1926.
9. Goodnow, M.: Nursing history, ed. 9, Philadelphia, 1955, W. B. Saunders Co.
10. Gubert, S.: Nurses in Italy, Nursing Mirror, **140**(4):63-66, 1975.
11. Huttenback, M.: A semester in Italy, Nursing Forum **5:**74-83, 1966.
12. Jameison, E., Sewall, M., and Suhrie, E.: Trends in nursing history, ed. 6, Philadelphia, 1966, W. B. Saunders Co.
13. Jensen, D. M.: History and trends in professional nursing, St. Louis, 1955, The C. V. Mosby Co.
14. Nutting, M. A., and Dock, L. L.: A history of nursing, Vol. 4, New York, 1910, G. P. Putnam's Sons.
15. Saunders, R. G.: Nursing and social services in Italy, Nursing Mirror **85:**193-195, June 15, 1947.
16. Seymer, L.: A general history of nursing, London, 1935, Faber & Faber Ltd.
17. Sgarra, A.: Organization of the nursing profession in Italy, International Nursing Review **2:**48-54, April, 1955.
18. Sgarra, A.: The nursing profession in Italy, Nursing Mirror **105:**1957-1959, 1957.
19. Stewart, I., and Austin, A.: A history of nursing, Philadelphia, 1962, G. P. Putnam's Sons.

Chapter 8

GREECE

EARLY NURSING IN GREECE

In Greece the transition from medieval to modern professional nursing was brought about by Roman Catholic and Eastern Orthodox religious orders and later through the influence of the Red Cross.[15] Some changes were effected by deaconesses, but they carried little significance because of the relative unimportance of Protestantism in Greece. Late in the nineteenth century, Queen Olga took an interest in nursing and established a two-year training school for nurses. In 1885 the Evangelismos Hospital was founded for the training of students.[3]

Queen Sophia had a similar interest in the professions, and hence in 1914 a two-year training school was established for student volunteers and put under the direction of the Red Cross.[3] Graduates of these schools contributed to the establishment of the Greek Red Cross School of Nursing and Public Health Nursing in Athens in 1924.[3] As the preceding statements suggest, the profession of nursing in Greece owes part of its development to the vital support of the Royal family.

Public health work started in Greece as early as 1919 and took place in baby welfare stations under the auspices of the Patriotic League of Social Welfare and Assistance and with the help of the American Red Cross.[2,9] In the beginning the workers were volunteers, but on establishment of the Greek Red Cross School of Nursing, more emphasis was put on the training of public health nurses.[2]

The Red Cross School of Nursing was the first school in Greece that was founded on a modern basis by operating a three-year program—a time frame that was internationally accepted at that time.[3,16] Student nurses, who numbered about thirty each year, took the schools' final examination, which was virtually a state examination. The school was directed by Athena Messolora, a Red Cross graduate who had taken a postgraduate course in public health nursing in London.[3] Her contributions to the development of nursing in Greece and her leadership role as a school director make her professional career outstanding in the nursing history of Greece.

The Kokina School of Nursing at Piraeus was started in 1927 by the American Women's Association and was attached to the American Women Hospital. It offered a three-year course in nursing under the administration of the American-Trained Nurse, an association of American nurses in Greece.[3,16] Students of this school, who were mainly refugees from Asia Minor, took the same final examination that the Red Cross School of Nursing offered.[16] Only twenty-seven nurses were graduated from this school before it had to close in 1933 for lack of funding and facilities.[3]

The Near East Foundation, in its program on rural and refugee camp work in 1930, trained many women in home health care and care of the sick. Trainees from this program did excellent work in helping during wars and in combatting infectious diseases in peacetime.[1]

Four graduate nurses from the Greek Red Cross School of Nursing helped in the reorganization of the Evangelismos Hospital School of Nursing, and as a result of their efforts the school started a three-year course for nurse training in 1930.[4] In 1935 the Model Health Center was established following an agreement between the City of Athens, the School of Hygiene, and the Rockefeller Foundation. The center was intended to be a training and demonstration health facility for public health students and for student nurses in the Red Cross and the Evangelismos Hospital School of Nursing. Students were required to spend two months at the center as part of their training.[4] A six-months' postbasic course was also offered by the Model Health Center for graduate nurses who wished to work in the community. With the outbreak of World War II, the center had to suspend operations.

An institution that combined hospital and public health nursing within a three-year period was established in 1938 and was known as the State School of Nursing and Public Health Nursing. Students joining this program were subjected to university entrance requirements.[4] Since 1948, and by a Royal decree, all students entering the three-year program in a school of nursing must meet the same university entrance requirements.[4]

In 1946 a military nursing school with a three-year program was established to meet the army nursing needs. In addition, the old Greek Red Cross Volunteer Nursing School was still active in preparing volunteer nurses in a six-month course to serve in war or natural disasters. Schools for nurses' aides, public health, and practical nurses were started during the war in an attempt to meet the country's evergrowing needs for nurses. After the war only three schools with a one-year training program were still training the practical nurses who were functioning in hospitals.[4]

NURSING EDUCATION IN GREECE

The overall nursing education program in Greece follows requirements set by the Ministry of Health for all schools of nursing.[10] The basic and fundamental objective is the correlation of theory with practice. Students obtain their theoretical instruction in medical and surgical nursing, obstetrics, pediatrics, psychiatry, and public health nursing at the time they are receiving their clinical experience in the corresponding fields in various hospitals and public health agencies. Public health has been integrated in all the courses throughout the students' experience.[10] The education of midwives is conducted separately in Greece. At present three schools for midwifery offer three-year programs.

Students in all schools of nursing pay no tuition fees, since all education is free in Greece. They receive free board and lodging, but they do not receive stipends. All students have to sit for a final examination conducted by their respective school's examining board. No state examination is available; however, the diploma is confirmed by the Ministry of Social Affairs, and the new graduates are registered in the Nursing Education Department of the ministry. To be licensed, all registered nurses in Greece must serve for three years after graduation in a state institution.[12]

Today, nine schools of nursing exist in Greece, three of them having a combined program of general and public health nursing. Of the nine, four are independent institutions affiliated with various health agencies to provide field experience for their students, whereas the rest are attached to hospitals. Eight of these schools are located in Athens and one in Thessalonika. Three are state schools, one is operated by the Red Cross, one by the Patriotic League of Social Welfare, and four by hospitals.[11-13]

NURSING ORGANIZATION

In 1923 the Hellenic National Graduate Nurses' Association was founded in Greece through the efforts of eleven nurses who were trained abroad. Later, graduates of the Hellenic Red Cross School of Nursing joined the association, which became a member of the International Council of Nurses in 1929. The association presently edits a bimonthly nursing journal, *Hellilis Adelphi* (Hellenic Nurse), which is active in raising the standards of nursing in the country.[11,12]

NURSING LEGISLATION

The first nursing section in the Ministry of Social Welfare was established in 1947 with Helen Petralia as chief nurse.[11] Recognition of the Nursing Bureau at the ministry by the Parliament took place in 1948, and a Nursing Legislation Act was passed that placed nursing education and registration under its supervision.[11] Thus nursing as a profession was given its rightful place among other professions. Graduate nurses were recognized by law as First Level Civil Employees, at present granting them equal rank with all other university graduates. The Nursing Bureau developed a unified educational program, and supervisory committees were established to check if schools of nursing were carrying out the right schedule of study. The Nursing Bureau, in addition, defined conditions of service, rank, promotion, and salaries—all major issues facing nurses at the time.

REFERENCES

1. Carr, A.: Nursing in pre-war Greece, American Journal of Nursing **42:**370-372, 1942.
2. Dock, L., and Stewart, I.: A short history of nursing, New York, 1938, G. P. Putnam's Sons.
3. Griffin, E., and Griffin, J.: Jensen's history and trends of professional nursing, St. Louis, 1969, The C. V. Mosby Co.
4. Ledakis, S.: Nursing education in Greece, International Nursing Review **4:**49-54, Jan., 1957.
5. McCarrick, H.: Aristotle's midwife, Nursing Times **66:**1470-1471, 1970.
6. Messolora, A.: Some aspects of nursing in Greece, American Journal of Nursing **40:**635-636, 1940.
7. Messolora, A.: Athena Messolora, International Nursing Review **12:**70-71, Nov. 12, 1965.
8. Nicolo, S.: O. R. nursing in Greece, AORN Journal **19:**114-120, 1974.
9. Noyes, L.: Establishment of foreign training schools, American Journal of Nursing **19:**947-948, 1919.
10. Papamicrouli, S.: The Greek Red Cross School for nurses and public health nurses, International Nursing Review **10:**29, Oct., 1963.
11. Papamicrouli, S.: Nursing in Greece, International Nursing Review **14:**25-28, May-June, 1967.
12. Papamicrouli, S.: Hellenic Red Cross School of Nursing: a combined program in general and public health nursing, International Journal of Nursing Studies **6:**27-35, 1969.
13. Papamicrouli, S.: Nursing in Greece, Journal of Psychiatric Nursing **7:**140-142, 1969.
14. Rosaria, L.: Nurse and child in Greek life, Journal of Pediatrics **30:**205-213, 1947.
15. Sellew, G., and Ebel, E.: A history of nursing, ed. 3, St. Louis, 1955, The C. V. Mosby Co.
16. Seymer, L.: A general history of nursing, London, 1935, Faber & Faber Ltd.
17. Smith, M.: American public health methods in the Near East, American Journal of Nursing **28:**463-465, 1928.

Chapter 9

NORTHERN EUROPE

The deaconess movement of Kaiserwerth, Germany, influenced nursing in Norway, Sweden, Iceland, Denmark, and Finland, as it did in all countries where Lutheranism became dominant after the Protestant reform.[19] When the Red Cross prepared for hospital nurse training in 1864 in Northern Europe, its promoters looked to Florence Nightingale for advice. As a result, a Swedish student, Emmy Rapp, was sent to St. Thomas's School of Nursing for training. On her return to Sweden, she directed the schools of nursing in Red Cross hospitals. Emmy Rapp was regarded as Sweden's first trained nurse and a path breaker for many others who followed.[7]

Since a similar pattern in nursing development and practice exists among the Northern European countries, special reference will be made to Sweden only with the hope that the reader will transpose the development of nursing in this country to other countries in the region.

Sweden

Systematic training of nurses began in Sweden in 1884 and originated from the initiative of Queen Sophia, who cherished a desire to provide regular instruction in nursing based on Christian principles.[13] This stimulated the establishment of the Sophia Home, or the Sophiahemmet Hospital, in 1889, which offered a training course in nursing to selected candidates.[25] In 1901 the South of Sweden Nursing Home was opened to train nurses for hospital and private nursing in southern Sweden.[13] The Sophiahemmet was built primarily to give nurses a source of practical training and at the same time a house for their residence during the two-year training period. Student nurses received no stipends. They were required to pay tuition for their training—an uncommon situation in Europe at the time.[2,14] In 1905 most schools were offering a three-year course in nursing.[14,20]

STATE INVOLVEMENT

Up to 1920 the state took little interest in nursing, but in that year Parliament passed several acts that provided state registration of nurses, state supervision of nursing education, and state-controlled employment bureaus for nurses. This action proved to be successful from the viewpoint of the public and the nurse, giving protection to both.[2] A nursing division was established at the same time under the Royal Board of Health with Kerstin Nordendahl, a graduate of the Sophiahemmet, as its head. As a result, many small nursing schools had to close, since they did not fulfill the requirements set by the board. They included stipulations specifying that no school could be opened without a board permit, and board approval of the teaching plan of every school was necessary, after which the institution remained under state supervision.[2]

NURSING ASSOCIATION

The Swedish Nurses' Association, which was founded in 1910 with Emmy Lindhagen as first president, was concerned mainly with developments in nursing education.[12] The question of salaries, employment, and working conditions was left to the nursing division of the Royal Board of Health. Since 1917 postgraduate courses in hospital administration and teaching have been offered by the association.[2] In 1933 the association adopted the *Swedish Journal of Nursing* as a private enterprise.[2] In addition to promoting the development of nursing so that the needs of all the people will be served best, the Swedish Nurses' Association takes an active interest in legislation affecting hospital construction, in emerging health care fields, and in vocational guidance. It is also influential in matters of general education and social issues, which were supported by Gerda Hojer, a Swedish nurse of international reputation who served as the president of the International Council of Nurses in 1947.[11]

Because of the similarity of the Scandinavian languages, Nordic congresses could be established, literature exchanged, study tours arranged, and nurses interchanged among hospitals of the different countries. This has kept the various nursing associations in close contact with each other and has led to the development of a regional organization known as the Association of Northern European Nurses. It meets in convention every four years. This allowed for more exchange of ideas among nurses and has stimulated interest among student nurses of one country to take nursing courses in another.[11]

THE SWEDISH FEDERATION

In January, 1965, a new federation was organized in Sweden on the initiative of the Swedish Nurses' Association. This newly founded association was called the Swedish Federation of Salaried Employees in Hospital and Public Health Services, which included, beside the Nurses' Association, the Laboratory Technicians Association, and the Medical Technology Association.[16] The main task of the federation was to work for improved salary and employment conditions and to support the newly developing fields in technology in legal matters until they could stand on their own feet.[8,16] The Swedish Nurses' Association has a long history of continuous effort in the development of bargaining rights for nurses and others belonging to the federation. Much of the collective bargaining done in Sweden then was based on practice rather than legislation until 1936, when a law was passed that recognized the association as the negotiating body between employer and employee. Since 1966 all public service officials are covered by an act that permits nurses to resort to strike action if negotiations fail.[4]

NURSING EDUCATION

All activities in the fields of public health and hospital care in Sweden are either operated or controlled by public authorities. The Ministry of Health and Social Affairs is responsible for the health services at the governmental level. The National Board of Health and Welfare governs, superintends, and promotes the activities and work of the institutions in the field. In other words, the board supervises the medical personnel, the hospitals, and the pharmacies and grants licensure to physicians, registered nurses, midwives, and other medical personnel.[17]

Before 1968 all nurses underwent a three-year education program, which included a certain amount of specialization in one or two branches that was given in the third year of study. In 1966 nursing education was recognized, and a new curriculum was established, comprising two and one-half years of study, at the end of which registration could be achieved. The program provides the students with a broad educational background in nursing, after which they are qualified as general nurses in any hospital. Specialization is now offered after registration in fields such as pediatrics, operating room, and midwifery.[1,15]

Sweden has thirty-four nursing schools, that have the same organization, syllabus, and curriculum. Nursing education at present is free of charge, and nursing students receive scholarships and financial aid from the government.[10,17] The trend now is to establish combined schools for training in various health fields, for example, basic nursing education, post-basic nursing education, practical nursing education, nurses' aide education, x-ray and laboratory technician education, and others. Many schools of nursing are presently housed in such facilities.[17]

Requirements for admission to a school of nursing include a minimum age of 18 years and the completion of ninth grade of the compulsory school leaving certificate. The length of basic nursing education is five semesters of twenty-one weeks each, during which theory and practice in medical-surgical, pediatrics, obstetrics, public health, and psychiatric nursing are given. A diploma is awarded at the end of the program, which entitles the nurse to state registration.[17,23]

In 1968 a general pattern of postbasic education was proposed in a government bill that established curricula in different fields in a program of one or two semesters, depending on the specialty. These curricula are established for the following fields of study:

Medical and surgical nursing	1 semester
Geriatric nursing	1 semester
Psychiatric nursing	1 semester
Anesthesiology nursing	2 semesters
Operating room nursing	2 semesters
Intensive care nursing	2 semesters
Pediatric nursing	2 semesters
Maternity and gynecological nursing (nurse-midwifery)	2 semesters
Public health nursing	2 semesters

The aim of the program is to prepare professional nurses for leadership positions. Requirements for admission include state registration and an employment period that ranges between six months for all the fields and two years for public health nurses.[17,21]

Advanced nursing education is offered at the State Institute of Advanced Nursing Education, headquartered in Stockholm, and four other branches in different parts of the country. Courses in nursing education are fifty-six weeks long, and nursing service administration covers a forty-week period. Requirements for admission to both programs include state registration, two years of experience, and meeting the university entrance requirements.[17]

Training for practical nurses was started in 1962. The practical nursing course requires thirty-two weeks, or twenty-three weeks if the student has at least one year of experience as an aide. A course for nurses' aides is also offered and is twenty-three weeks long with no educational requirement.[10] Practical nurses in general hospital wards, operating rooms, or outpatient departments may take up registered nurse training in a course that has been shortened from five semesters to three semesters, acknowledging their previously acquired knowledge.[24] (See Fig. 5.)

Midwifery training in Sweden is changing to fit in with the new general nursing scheme. Student nurses in midwifery are required to complete the two- and one-half–year training course before they go into midwifery. Training will then take one academic year, during which many medical procedures are practiced. At present, two midwifery schools are available in Sweden, since the national policy is to centralize courses.[10]

The jobs of health visitor and district nurse in Sweden are combined

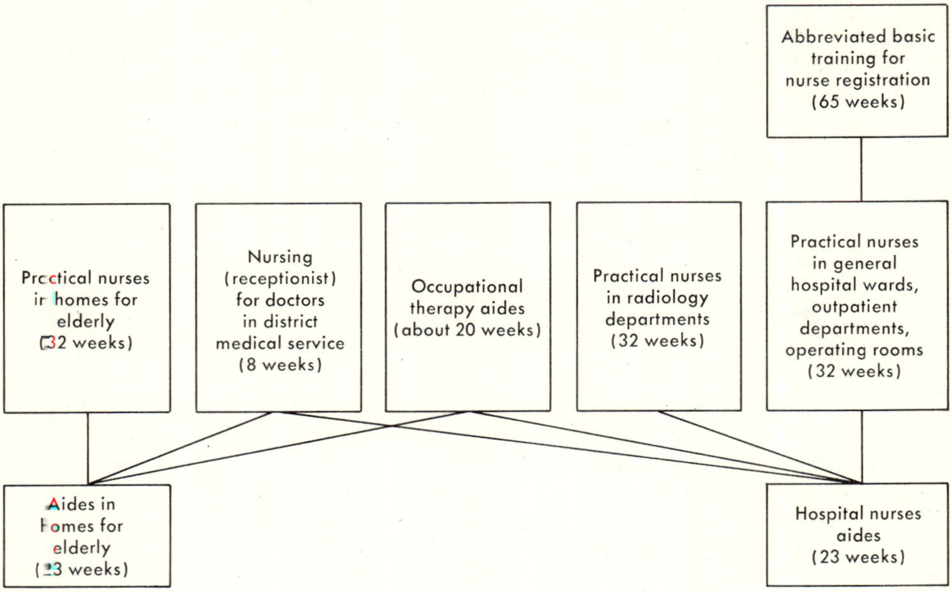

FIG. 5

Auxiliary nursing personnel. (Modified from Training of auxiliary nursing personnel, Stockholm, 1974, The National Swedish Board of Education.)

and carried out by one individual. Two public health nurse–training centers are in existence, and students receive state grants during their training and work alongside the physicians.[5] Although little public health nursing is available in Sweden compared with that offered in other countries, home help nursing services are always available to families who need them. These are provided through the training of women as home nurses, who are constantly supervised by the few public health nurses.[10]

HEALTH CARE IN SWEDEN

In Sweden the main administration of health care services is controlled by the local authorities—the Regional Councils—that are responsible for the planning, day-to-day financing, and organizing of hospitals. The emphasis is on intermediate care at the community level; this was believed to be an economical way of providing better care to the patient. The emphasis on hospital care now is decreasing, and the patient is increasingly oriented to the local health center, which usually has general practitioners, nurses, social workers, and sometimes specialists who offer individualized patient care. Localized personal documentation ensured that medical records are easily available—an important aspect of community care that saves time, transport, and travel and provides a better and more personal service to the individual.[6]

An important feature of the Swedish health centers is their affiliation with nursing homes that treat chronically and physically sick patients. Some health centers are deeply involved in research in addition to providing personalized care to patients. Others are attached to hospitals that provide specialist outpatient care as a measure to take the burden off the hospital and outpatient department in offering specialist advice and care.[9]

The provision of specialized care by the health center has contributed to the development and expansion of the nurse's role. Nurses are given courses locally in different specialty areas, such as diabetes and cancer, and are asked to attend classes for medical students at a local university before taking over the management of the specialty clinics. The nurses are responsible for the medical history, physical examination, assessment of the patient's condition, and follow-up care. The physician checks on the patient once a year only and when the patient is referred to the physician by the nurse.[6] This new role is welcomed by the nurses in Sweden as well as by other authorities that are demanding more specialization and training of nurses.

All the rest of the Northern European countries enjoy a socialized health care delivery system that is more or less similar to the Swedish system. The development of nursing in all of them follows a pattern. All countries share a common belief that the function of the professional nurse cannot remain static. Qualified nurses are expected to have more technical and increased responsibilities when working in specialized units. It is hoped that this trend will bring about expansion in the nurse's role.

COMMUNITY NURSING IN THE HEALTH CARE DELIVERY SYSTEM

A modern health care delivery system requires for its functioning a trained body of health professionals. When the health needs of a society change, a mechanism should go into operation, rearranging the work done by the different professionals. This should also be accompanied by an adaptation in the training of the different kinds of health professionals. One benefit from such a change is the need for an interaction between the educational and health care delivery systems of the country.[18]

In October, 1974, a shortage of public health personnel existed in Sweden, including physicians and public health nurses.[24] However, the number of nurses has increased considerably since then, especially in the public health section. Community health nursing seems to be the trend in Sweden. This group of professionals carry on outpatient work outside the hospital. Their functions include preventive health care, medical care, and sociomedical care. At present 3,000 community health nurses and 400 district midwives are employed in the Swedish community services. These employees have three years of undergraduate nursing, two years of practical experience, and one year of specialization training.[3]

Community health nursing in Sweden forms a major part of the primary health care delivery system. The goals of this system include providing comprehensive health care, local services and easy accessibility, continuity of care, and reliability and quality of services. These goals are enhanced by interaction among the different branches of the health care delivery system. Preventive health care, curative health care, sociomedical care, and other administrative duties comprise the functions of a community health nurse in such a system. These tasks are expected to increase as new techniques and facilities are developed in the health care arena.

Organizationally, the work in a community health center is divided among community health nurses, midwives, pediatric nurses, physiotherapists, occupational therapists, junior nurses and nurses' aides, district medical officers, social workers, office clerks, and domestic aid supervisors. In general, community health nursing should be built around the largest health care center in the primary care area, where local centers could be attached for local service.

The health care delivery system in Sweden functions as an organic whole, with a defined relationship between its different institutions and levels of medical care. A unique feature of such a system is the fact that the local communities direct almost all of the system through a decentralized regional organization, and the overall national coordination is achieved by voluntary contact and orderly advice from government officials but with little government domination.

REFERENCES

1. Adler, S. P.: Swedish student nurses: a descriptive study, Nursing Research **18:**363-365, 1969.
2. Andrell, M.: Nursing in Sweden, American Journal of Nursing **40:**1336-1341, 1940.
3. Axelsson, S., and Nicolausson, U.: Community health nursing—farthest outpost of the health and medical services, Current Sweden **144:**1-7, 1977.
4. Bergkvist, G.: Collective bargaining in Sweden, International Nursing Review **15**(4):67-74, 1968.
5. Berglind, H.: Occupation activity of a Swedish RN, International Journal of Nursing Studies **2:**251-260, 1965.
6. Cawford, L.: Health care in Denmark, Sweden, and Holland, Nursing Mirror **141**(14):65-67, 1975.
7. Dock, L., and Stewart, I.: A short history of nursing, New York, 1938, G. P. Putnam's Sons.
8. Dunbar, V.: Nursing in Northern Europe, American Journal of Nursing **37:**123-130, 1937.
9. Hjern, B. O.: What about socialized medicine in Sweden? Archives of Surgery **111:**941-944, 1976.

10. Hooper, J.: Nurse training in Sweden, Aug., 1968, Nursing Times **65:**73-76, 1969.
11. Jameison, E., Sewall, M., and Suhrie, E.: Trends in nursing history, ed. 6, Philadelphia, 1966, W. B. Saunders Co.
12. Nordendahl, K.: Nursing in Sweden, American Journal of Nursing **48:**694-696, 1948.
13. Nutting, M. A., and Dock, L. L.: A history of nursing, Vol. 4, New York, 1910, G. P. Putnam's Sons.
14. Olsen, M.: Nursing in Sweden, American Journal of Nursing **32:**1059-1063, 1932.
15. Peck, L.: Psychiatric nursing in Sweden, Nursing Mirror **129:**27, Aug. 29, 1969.
16. Rabo, M.: Sweden initiating a new Federation, International Nursing Review **12:**34-36, Oct., 1965.
17. Rabo, M.: Nursing in Sweden, International Nursing Review **18**(4):334-348, 1971.
18. Rexed, B.: The role of medical education in planning the development of a national health care system, Journal of Medical Education **49:**27-42, 1974.
19. Sellew, G., and Ebel, E.: A history of nursing, ed. 3, St. Louis, 1955, The C. V. Mosby Co.
20. Setzler, L.: Stockholm diary, American Journal of Nursing **46:**46-47, 1946.
21. Swedish Board of Education: The postbasic nursing education in Sweden, 1970. Unpublished manuscript. (Available from the Royal Swedish Embassy, Washington, D.C.)
22. Swedish Board of Education: Training of auxiliary nursing personnel, 1974. Unpublished manuscript. (Available from the Royal Swedish Embassy, Washington, D.C.)
23. Swedish Board of Education: The basic nursing education in Sweden, 1975. Unpublished manuscript. (Available from the Royal Swedish Embassy, Washington, D.C.)
24. Swedish Institute: The organization of medical care, Fact Sheets on Sweden, 1976.
25. Wald, L.: The Sophiahemmet in Stockholm, American Journal of Nursing **1:** 180-182, 1900.

Chapter 10

YUGOSLAVIA

Yugoslavia is a federation comprising the republics of Serbia, Croatia, Slovenia, Montenegro, Bosnia, and Macedonia. The country has existed as a geographical and political entity since 1918, prior to which the republics were separate kingdoms. This has contributed to the unique lines along which nursing in Yugoslavia has developed.[3] The first developments in nursing are traced to 1856, when the government gave an order that all care of the sick in hospitals was to be undertaken by the Sisters of Charity.[7] This important event affected the development of nursing in the different republics.

EARLY NURSING PRACTICES

Except for the building of hospitals and the transfer of the sick from monasteries where they received treatment, no significant changes were noted between 1856 and World War I. At the end of the war, the revival of nursing and medical practices occurred as a result of war experiences and activities.[5] Numerous health centers were opened by the government to meet the urgent needs of postwar conditions. In 1919 the Slovania Faculty of Medicine was founded by the University of Ljubljana, which had important influences on the health services of the area. The same period also witnessed the arrival of the first registered nurse, Slovina Angela Boshin from Vienna.[5] Having been educated in Vienna under the Blue Sisters, she came to Yugoslavia to start the hard elementary work involved in the establishment of district nursing and social health. In 1924 a district nursing school was opened, which began by offering a one-year course.[7] Two other schools of nursing were established at about the same time. One is the Belgrade Training School for Nurses, which was started on the English plan in 1921 by Emid Newton. The other was the State School of Zaghreb, which trained students from both religious and secular orders.[5]

During the organization period in Yugoslavia, nursing had the support of Dr. Andrija Stampar, Director of Health and one of the outstanding public health leaders of Europe. His interest in community health was reflected in the training of public health nurses of the different schools. Because of Dr. Stampar's interest in welfare institutions, all schools of nursing and health centers stressed the concept of preventive care.[5,6]

DEVELOPMENT OF PROFESSIONAL NURSING

Professional nursing experienced a relatively slow development until 1945. However, after World War II, nursing developed rapidly. Factors that influenced its progress were the shortage of nurses during and after the war and the rapid development of the country's health services with increased governmental interest in nursing.[10] In each republic, councils of health and social policy were established that were responsible for setting up schools of nursing and determining the regulations under which they should be conducted.[10] As a result, three types of schools were started, which varied in academic level, admission requirements, and length of the course. An advanced school of nursing offered a three-year program in which applicants had to meet the university entrance requirements. A middle medical school also offered a three-year program but admitted students with only four years of high school. The third school offered a program that also required students to have completed four years of high school.[10]

The advanced schools of nursing were established in 1951. The one in Belgrade was administered by the Red Cross Committee of Yugoslavia. The curriculum of all schools of nursing prepared students for both hospital and public health work.[9] Until 1950, no postgraduate course of study was available to graduate nurses in Yugoslavia except for the programs offered at the schools for midwives. But since then postgraduate courses have been offered in teaching, head nursing, operating room nursing, nurse dietetics, and public health nursing.

NURSING ASSOCIATION

The nurses' association in Yugoslavia is a Federation of Nurses' Association of the Republics of Slovenia, Croatia, Macedonia, and Servia. The Yugoslavian Graduate Nurses' Association was established in 1926 by the graduates of the first school of nursing in Zaghreb, and in 1929 the association became affiliated with the International Council of Nurses. In 1931 an act signed by the king provided for the three-year curricula, set standards for admission, established proper selection and organization of nursing faculty, and defined the status of nurses.[8]

After World War II the nurses in each republic began to reform their own branches of the association. The federation was admitted into membership with the International Council of Nurses in 1957, since it had dropped out after the Communist revolution.[7,8] The different associations were active at the district level, where seminars, refresher courses, and postgraduate programs were offered to nurses in different fields.

NURSING EDUCATION

A brief explanation of the general education system in Yugoslavia may be helpful in understanding the nursing education system. All students in this Eastern European country attend elementary school for eight years, after which they *may* enter a four-year middle school, which combines general education with training for a technical, vocational, or semiprofessional career. Basic nursing education is included in this program. On the other hand, students *may* choose to enter a four-year academic school *(Gimnazija)*, at the completion of which they can enter the university or an advanced school that prepares them for special careers. The three-year advanced nursing course is included in this program.[1] (See Fig. 6.)

In 1963 the Advanced School of Public Health was established by the Yugoslavia Red Cross Society. It trains teachers and administrators for

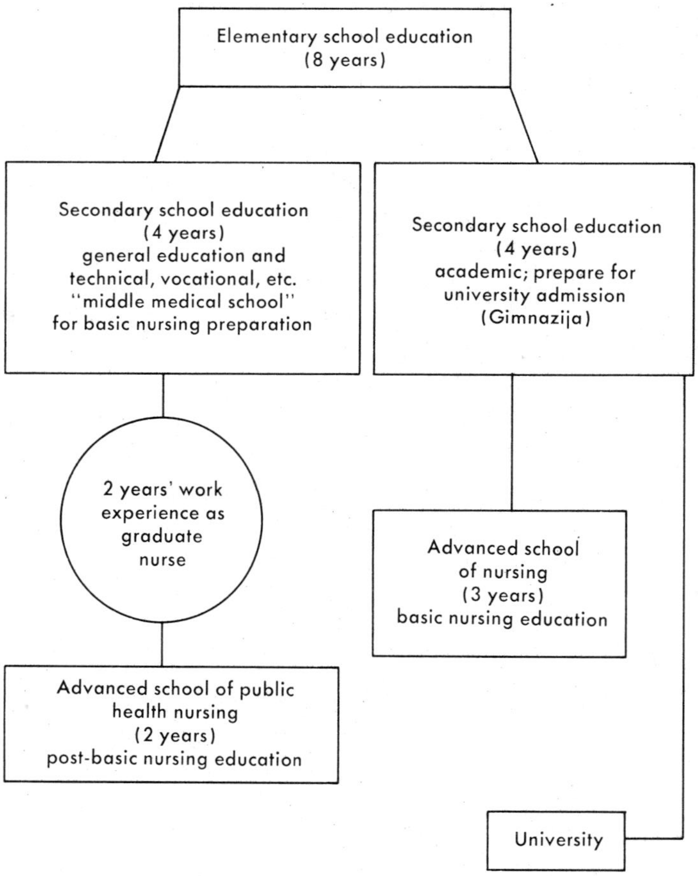

FIG. 6

Nursing education in Yugoslavia. (Modified from Benson, E.: Nursing Outlook **17:** 36-38, 1969.)

public health leadership positions in a two-year program. To be admitted, a student should have completed the middle school nursing program and should have worked as a nurse for at least two years.[2]

Training for midwivery and pediatric nursing is available in Yugoslavia at present, and the program covers four years. Middle school nursing is now expanded to cover four years instead of three. Many advanced schools that require applicants to meet university admission standards have been established and are gaining in popularity. A program that offers a two-year course to train assistant nurses, whose duties are similar to those of licensed practical nurses in the United States, is now available also.[1] Schools of nursing at all levels are approved by the Councils of Health in each republic. In addition, a state examination is set by the Central Council of Health; the grading of the salary scales depends on the passing of this examination.[4]

Since a great similarity exists in the health care systems among the Eastern European countries, the reader will find them operating more or less along the same line. Differences do exist, however, between those countries with roots in Communist patterns that dominate the health care delivery system in Eastern Europe and those countries of the Western World. In spite of the restraints, Yugoslavia and Poland have shown greater initiative than neighboring countries in their attempt to unite with nurses in the world and in the improvement of nursing education and service.[11]

The summary of nursing education in Yugoslavia can perhaps best be illustrated by consulting Fig. 6.

REFERENCES

1. Benson, E.: Vignette of nursing in Yugoslavia, Nursing Outlook **17:**36-38, 1969.
2. Benson, E.: Nurse to nurse contact on the international scene. International Nursing Review **18**(3):281-286, 1971.
3. Benson, E.: Nursing in Serbia . . . early days, American Journal of Nursing **74:** 472-474, 1974.
4. Bridges, D.: Yugoslavia, International Nursing Review **6:**23-27, Jan., 1959.
5. Dock, L., and Stewart, I.: A short history of nursing, New York, 1938, G. P. Putnam's Sons.
6. Ingram, R.: Nursing in Yugoslavia, American Journal of Nursing **30:**139-145, 1930.
7. Slovenija, S. E.: The development of nursing in Northern Yugoslavia, International Journal of Nursing Studies **9:**151-158, 1972.
8. Some impressions of nursing in Yugoslavia and Hungary, American Journal of Nursing **31:**671-676, 1931.
9. Stewart, I., and Austin, A.: A history of nursing, New York, 1962, G. P. Putnam's Sons.
10. Urbancic, D.: Nursing in Yugoslavia, American Journal of Nursing **56:**585-587, 1956.
11. White, K. L.: International comparisons of medical care utilization, New England Journal of Medicine **277:**516-522, 1967.

Chapter 11

RUSSIA

In Russia the development of the nursing profession followed a unique pattern, and whether it was ever influenced by the British system is doubtful. The Sisters of Mercy in Russia existed as far back as the Crimean War, but they were different from the religious orders of the Catholic countries.[6] These sisters were voluntary workers who came from upper class families or were widows of army officers.[6,20] In Russia the Red Cross was preeminent in nursing, and Red Cross nurses were trained in a two-year hospital course following the German and Scandinavian Red Cross patterns.[16] Until then, nursing services that involved cleanliness and the comfort of the patient were performed by servants.[5,9] The Russian word for a nurse is *sestra* (sister). It was first used by the Red Cross nurses who belonged at the beginning to a submedical rather than a nursing class because they were employed chiefly for doing dressings and treatments.[5,6,20] As early as the 1870s, women started studying medicine and achieved high status in the profession, since in Russia intellectual equality for men and women was recognized and professional study by women was greatly encouraged.[6]

THE RUSSIAN REVOLUTION

The revolution of 1917 and the radical changes that followed wiped out most of the old order, and under the new Communist government an entirely new system of medical and health care was established. The class structure was changed, with workers given first appointments in educational fields and work. A system of secular ethics was introduced that called for complete subordination of the individual to the authority of the state.[20]

A unique feature of the Russian system was the adoption of a nationwide health scheme based on the health needs and resources of the country. This resulted in a five-year plan, which was subsequently divided into quotas for every field, with the military services having first precedence. Many women were assigned to medical and health services, and many educated men who belonged to the upper class were drafted as officers and engineers in the army.[20]

Medical practice was reorganized into lower, middle, and higher levels, establishing a three-step vocational ladder that separated the unskilled from the skilled workers and the skilled and semiprofessionals from the professionals.[4] No strict lines were drawn between the different levels designed to allow for mobility of workers from one rung to another, provided they qualified by additional preparation and experience. The government also identified a shortage of nurses and the great need for their services, resulting in the establishment of many schools of nursing that offered short courses in an attempt to train nurses. Later, many *fledshers* (physician's assistants), both men and women, received a three-year training course that prepared them to become physician's assistants. This group of nurses was allowed to do minor surgery and prescribe medicine.[8]

Nurses, along with the *fledshers* and midwives, belonged to the middle medical category. On the lowest level were the aides and orderlies who had some practical training after the four years of general education. Physicians belonged to the highest level.[4] Many women physicians in Russia had taken nursing or midwifery training before they went into medicine. This makes the nursing profession a halfway house among other career levels and also explains the lack of leaders in the nursing field.[4,8] In other words, nursing preparation was considered to be a step toward qualifying as a physician.

Since all the health work was done by the government in Russia, which was, in a sense, in the field of public health, little distinction existed between the public health nurse and the institutional nurse. No private hospitals, private nurses, and private journals existed in Russia beside those which are government owned. The nurses were trained, employed, and paid by the state. The whole health system was controlled by the *Narkomzdrav*, or the Ministry of Public Health, which governed and determined nurses' training and practice. In 1935 the first law defining the title "nurse" was passed. It stipulated that only graduate nurses of a recognized hospital training school of nursing who passed the final examination could be considered nurses.[2] Through the enactment of this law, nursing became a profession with defined duties and responsibilities. Nursing education witnessed the integration of theory and practice and the setting of admission requirements for all candidates applying to enter the nursing schools.[2]

All nursing programs started with a two-year program, at the end of which a certificate was issued.[17] Specialty areas in midwifery, public health, and pediatric nursing were available in a one-year course for graduate nurses who achieved outstanding results in the final examination.[10] The two-year graduate in Russia always worked as an assistant to the physician,[10] whereas the three-year graduate had more medical responsibilities and functioned on the same level as an intern in the United States.[10] The *fledsher* functioned only occasionally as a nurse in the hospital. Most frequently this group took responsibility in directing a collective or state farm district clinic, a rural health center, or a first-aid medical station in a mine or factory and in some places acting as a substitute for the physician.[7]

NURSING ORGANIZATION

With the establishment of the Communist regimes, all workers were required to join one large union, which includes all levels of health personnel. Unions in Russia differ from those in the western world in that they are not self-governing, since they are a part of the state machinery and subject to control by higher authorities. As a result, these unions are not allowed to bargain for better conditions and salaries or to resort to strike if negotiations fail. Their chief function is to stimulate production in industry and to work for the improvement of health care administration. Many types of discipline are employed by unions for offenses or incompetent work. Also, a system of honors was developed for good work and accepted Communist conduct.[20] Attendance at union meetings is compulsory, since all Russian citizens are supposed to do some voluntary social work through the unions as a contribution to the welfare of the general public.

All nurses are encouraged to participate in the local community and governmental organizations such as the Red Cross, Local Soviets, or other voluntary and governmental bodies. Professionally, beside membership in the medical workers union, nurses have attempted to organize themselves in a society for the pursuit of professional interests. The Moscow Bothin Hospital has had a Nursing Soviet Council since 1938. In 1958 the Ministry of Health described procedures for organizing similar councils on local hospital levels. This body of nurses was responsible for conducting programs in nursing as well as seminars on issues and problems facing the profession. Some councils acted as inspection groups that examined and evaluated the work of lower medical personnel.[7,14]

NURSING EDUCATION

At present in Russia a young man or women can enroll for training in a nursing school on the completion of eighth grade. The training requires three years; a high percentage of the curriculum comprises general education, and courses such as history, social science, literature, physics, chemistry, and a foreign language are offered. On completion of the program, students receive a general education certificate plus a tenth-grade certificate, which allow them to apply for university education.[1,18] However, students who have already finished ten years of secondary school skip the aforementioned subjects and go directly to the medical subjects, which include medical Latin, biology, anatomy and physiology, microbiology, pharmacy, hygiene, and health systems and administration. Special nursing subjects include care of internal and surgical diseases, anatomical and physiological peculiarities of children, care of children under 1 year of age, communicable diseases, nervous and psychiatric diseases, dermatological and venereal diseases, eye diseases, otolaryngological diseases, physiotherapy, physical culture, and pathology.[1]

No teaching is done by nurses. Basic courses are taught by the faculty from the respective social sciences departments. Physicians are responsible for the teaching of clinical subjects and for the training of nurses, which is provided in *oblast* (provincial) hospitals.[1] During the first year students' hospital experience emphasizes care of the environment. Patient care starts in the second year, during which students are taught to give injections and handle technical equipment. Throughout this period technical competency is emphasized. The third year provides students with an extensive practice period during which they rotate on different wards and prepare for the state examination. The head physician's recommendations of the students serve as a requirement for admission to the examination. At times the physician recommends additional study for the student to take before graduation.[1]

Training and distribution of medium-level medical personnel are conducted in accordance with the overall plan of development of the health service and extension of the network of medical colleges. In Russia, instruction is free, and hence the right to enter these colleges is enjoyed by all citizens under the age of 30 years. Entrance examinations must be passed before admission to the medical colleges. On graduation from the college, employment is provided to all in accordance with the distribution plan of the local health services.[12] As a general rule, all students who enter nursing schools in Russia are attracted to medicine. More than 20% of the graduate nurses, after a few years of experience, apply to medical schools to become physicians.[11,21] Nurses and physicians are obliged to take refresher courses of one to six months, depending on the area of specialty. Students in these courses are entitled to an allowance and living accommodations in addition to the salaries. Annual leaves with pay are also available to nurses interested in working in different areas as a measure of updating their knowledge.[21]

The training of a *fledsher* is similar to that of a nurse but requires six additional months for specialty training. Students in this group receive special preparation in first aid, diagnosis, and relatively independent practice under a physician's supervision. A graduate *fledsher* usually functions as an independent practitioner in a *fledsher* station. The midwifery training program is much the same as the *fledshers'* program but with emphasis on obstetrics rather than surgery. Practice is partly in general hospitals but mostly in maternity hospitals.[1]

Advanced nursing education as head nurses and anesthesiologists or as special surgical nurses is decided by the head physician who establishes whether a nurse is eligible for it. Two-year courses are offered at the Medical Education Institute in Moscow to nurses sponsored by the hospital administration. Further education for nurses covers areas such as physical therapy, surgery, obstetrics, pediatrics, psychiatry, and neurology. The number of nurses admitted to these programs depends on the kind of specialty training that the system requires.[1]

NURSING SERVICE

The present Russian medical plan emphasizes training of medical *sestras* (nurses) in a program that has advanced training in preventive care. The new medical practitioner and the medical *sestra* are then assigned as a team to work in a rural station. The *sestras* function in hospitals, polyclinics, and ambulatory health services and in this role serve as assistants to the physician.[1,13]

The chief physician in every Russian hospital is also the chief administrative officer. The chief nurse is directly responsible to the chief physician and essentially acts as his or her assistant. Senior nurses in different departments are automatically responsible to the senior physicians of the respective departments and work under their direct supervision. The senior physician and nurse work as a team to supervise the services provided in a unit. No nursing service department is available, and hence no direct line of authority exists between staff nurses and the chief nurse.[15] Russian nurses apparently do not believe in a nursing hierarchy, but instead, the physician, nurse, and auxiliary personnel work as a team with the physician in charge. This pattern also prevails in polyclinics and other health units, where duties are perceived as interchangeable.[15] It is of interest to note that the nursing profession is not reserved exclusively for women in Russia. Many male students join the nursing schools; however, most of them become *fledshers*.[21]

HEALTH SERVICES

In Russia the provision of health care is guaranteed by the state. No direct charges are made to the patient. All health services are unified, centrally directed, and accessible to all persons in need. The system is characterized by a degree of centralization of planning and direction at the national level and by decentralization of execution and implementation at the four lower levels. These are the fifteen republics, the *oblast* which is a province of the republic, the *rayon* which is a subdivision of the *oblast,* and the *uchastok,* or local district.[1] Each of the republics has a Ministry of Health; the *oblast* and *rayon* each has a health department that controls the *uchastok.*[1,3]

The hospital system includes the *uchastok* hospital, the *rayon* hospital, and the *oblast,* or city, hospital. The *punkt,* or station, is the smallest unit and is run by *fledshers* or midwives. It serves as the first contact point of the patient with the health care delivery system. Patients admitted to the *uchastok* hospital who need a specialist's attention are referred to either the *rayon* or the *oblast* hospital.[1,19]

The polyclinics are the heart of the Russian health care system, with prevention as their primary goal. All polyclinics have their own staff of medical specialists in addition to providing the public with various paramedical services. Physicians who serve in *uchastok* hospitals also have offices in the polyclinics. Vaccination, immunization, and follow-up care are provided by sanitary epidemiological centers, which are separate from the polyclinics. Considerable reliance is placed on these centers for improving and maintaining the health of the people. Some of these polyclinics are integrated with *rayon* or *oblast* hospitals, whereas others are independent and free standing.[1]

The nursing profession enjoys prestige in Russia; many nurses are elected to political offices. This is attributed to the heroic work done by nurses during World War II as well as to the competent and devoted work presently done at the various levels. The chief difficulty with the Russian system, however, is that it does not provide any real identification for nursing as a profession as separate from other fields. Instead, nursing acts as a halfway point on the professional ladder.

REFERENCES

1. Abdellah, F.: Nursing and health care in the USSR, American Journal of Nursing **73:**2096-2099, 1973.
2. Albin, E.: Nursing in the USSR, American Journal of Nursing **46:**525-528, 1946.
3. Armstrong, J.: Health services in the USSR, Nursing Times **61:**1592, 1965.
4. Bullough, V., and Bullough, B.: The emergence of modern nursing, ed. 2, London, 1969, The Macmillan Co.
5. Dock, L.: Hospital nursing in Russia, American Journal of Nursing **9:**755-757, 1909.
6. Dock, L., and Stewart, I.: A short history of nursing, New York, 1938, G. P. Putnam's Sons.
7. Ensberger, M.: Nursing in Russia, Nursing Outlook **11:**883, 1963.
8. Goodnow, M.: Nursing history, ed. 9, Philadelphia, 1955, W. B. Saunders Co.
9. Hoffman, I.: Progress in Russia, American Journal of Nursing **14:**197-198, 1913.
10. Holliday, J.: Glimpses of nursing in Russia, Nursing Outlook **6:**496-497, 1958.
11. Ikonnikova, J.: Nurses in the Soviet Union, International Nursing Review **10:** 17, July-Aug., 1963.
12. Kolylima, G.: Nursing in USSR, International Journal of Nursing Studies **4:**257, 1957.
13. Leitz, D.: Nursing in the Soviet Union, Nursing Mirror **117:**64-66, Jan. 31, 1964.

14. Morris, K. H.: Profile of a Russian nurse, American Journal of Nursing **66:**549-551, 1966.
15. Mussallem, K. H.: A glimpse of nursing in the USSR, Canadian Nurse **63:**27-33, 1967.
16. Noyes, C.: Establishment of foreign training school, American Journal of Nursing **19:**247-248, 1919.
17. Powell, A.: Journey to Moscow, Nursing Times **60:**481, 1964.
18. Powell, A.: Nurse training in USSR, Nursing Times **62:**1600-1601, 1966.
19. Quinn, S. E.: Nursing in the Soviet Union, International Nursing Review **15**(1): 75-86, 1968.
20. Stewart, I., and Austin, A.: A history of nursing, New York, 1962, G. P. Putnam's Sons.
21. Tarassova, G.: An honored profession, Nursing Times **69:**527-530, 1973.

PART III

The Americas

Chapter 12

CANADA

The development of nursing in Canada was influenced first by the religious orders who came from France to establish hospitals and homes for the sick, second by the Nightingale system and the Victorian Order of Nurses, and third by the United States, which has been responsible for the more recent developments. Modern Canadian nursing seems to be greatly influenced by the developments in United States nursing. On the other hand, Canada has furnished the United States with some of the outstanding leaders of the profession.[7,17]

The first Nightingale Schools of Nursing were started at about the same time in the United States and Canada. Dr. Theophilus Mack of the General and Marine Hospital in Ontario introduced the Nightingale nursing system to Canada in 1864 and later sent a Miss Money to London to study at St. Thomas's School in 1873. On her return a school of nursing was established in Toronto, and soon other hospital schools developed in larger cities. The Toronto General Hospital was the first to open in 1881 under Mary Agnes Snively, who had graduated from the Bellevue Hospital in New York. In 1890 the Montreal General Hospital School of Nursing was started under the leadership of Norah Livingston who was also a graduate of the Bellevue Hospital in New York. The history of Mary Agnes Snively and Norah Livingston mainly constitutes the history of nursing in Canada.[20,22] Graduates from both schools functioned in every part of Canada, building, developing, and reforming nursing schools.

The first school of nursing in the French Catholic Hospitals was at Nôtre Dame Hospital in Quebec, which was founded in 1899. Hôtel Dieu School of Nursing was then established in Montreal in 1901 and in 1920 was affiliated with the University of Montreal.[19] The Victorian Order of Nurses, a public health nursing service, was founded in 1897 by Lady Aberdeen. It provided services for all people in all districts and was expanded through the Lady Grey Country District Nursing Service in 1909 to include country districts in Canada.[7,19] Training involved different fields of study, preparing graduates to function as midwives, school nurses, and tuberculosis officers.[11,17]

THE CANADIAN RED CROSS

The organization of the Canadian Red Cross was founded in 1896 by Dr. George Sterling Ryerson. Prior to World War I the Red Cross societies confined their activities to war services, but during the war, efforts turned toward the prevention of communicable diseases. This resulted in the first mandate in Canada, which provided facilities for the postgraduate training of nurses in public health. For many years the Red Cross financed the employment in rural districts of public health nurses, whose main work concerned disease prevention and public education.[5]

In other respects the development of Canadian nursing has closely followed that of nursing in the United States. This was most obvious in the early affiliation with the university. In 1919 the first department of nursing at the university level was established as a result of the cooperation of the University of British Columbia and Vancouver General Hospital. Other schools were soon established in other universities, such as McGill University, University of Toronto, Nôtre Dame University, and the Universities of Manitoba and Alberta, which offered the bachelor's degree in nursing.

NURSING ORGANIZATIONS

The Canadian nurses were organized along lines similar to those of the American nurses. They had joined with those of the United States to form the American Society of Superintendents of Training Schools for nurses, founded in 1893 and followed in 1896 by the establishment of the Nurses Associated Alumni of the United States and Canada. Nurses from the associations were active in launching the first graduate program in nursing at Teacher's College, Columbia University, which opened in 1899.[22] Incidentally, the first two nurses to take a leading role in establishing the program, Isabel Hampton and Adelaide Nutting, were Canadian by nationality. The original associated alumni and the superintendents' societies encompassed both Canadian and United States nurses. This union split in 1907, and the Canadian National Association of Trained Nurses was formed.

As a result of the organization of the International Council of Nurses in 1899, Snively, acting as the organization's first treasurer, began a movement that led to the splitting of the United States–Canada associations and the formation of the Canadian Association of Nursing Education. This was done to achieve membership in the International Council of Nurses, which was then organized on a provisional basis, allowing only national nurses' associations to become members.[22]

In 1909 the Canadian Nurses' Association became the fourth member of the International Council of Nurses, and in 1922 nursing laws were secured in all the provinces. In 1924 the Nurses Associated Alumni of the United States and Canada and the Association of Nursing Education merged, resulting in what is now known as the Canadian Nurses' Association. The newly formed association had three sections: nursing education, private duty nursing, and public health nursing. In 1930 a federation of provincial associations was formed, each securing complete autonomy in dealing with its own problems.[7,22]

Similar to the American Nurses' Association, the Canadian Nurses' Association owned and controlled the *Canadian Nurse*, a journal established in 1910. Special mention should be made of Jean Wilson and Ethel Johns, who were instrumental in transforming the journal from an alumni quarterly to a national and then international publication.[7,22] The *Canadian Nurse* continued to develop and now publishes English and French editions that are widely distributed and respected throughout the world.

NURSING EDUCATION

The majority of nursing schools were operated by hospitals that provided students with free room, board, tuition, and, in some instance, a small monthly allowance in return for a substantial amount of service. That arrangement (students as a source of cheap labor for the hospitals) created a conflict and weakened the educational experience of students.[1]

However, by the end of World War I, Canadian universities opened their doors to nurses and those of McGill and Toronto started offering a one-year course for graduate nurses. McGill University was under the leadership of Flora Madelaine Shaw and Toronto University, under Kathleen Russel.[10] As was mentioned earlier, the first Canadian five-year program leading to a university degree was offered under the joint auspices of the University of British Columbia and the Vancouver General Hospital School of Nursing. The program was directed by Ethel Johns. These university programs were preceded by a centralized curriculum that was established to reduce duplication of courses in different schools of nursing. The Canadian Nurses' Association started this movement, which was later transferred to the different universities where lectures were given by the medical staff. Soon after the association's efforts to bring nursing to the university level were successful.[6]

As in most other countries, Canada had trained, partially trained, and untrained women whe engaged in practical nursing. In 1920, hospitals introduced an auxiliary staff of aides who worked in the wards under the direction of nurses. These were known as "nurses' aides." Their responsibilities were to assist nurses in performing simple duties associated with patient care. Later, another kind of auxiliary worker was introduced to the nursing scene—the certified assistant nurse. The student in this group was prepared under the direction of nurse instructors in schools financed by the government in a one-year training program.[3] The new emphasis on team nursing contributed to the development of the different levels of nurse preparation, placed nurses in leadership positions, and gave them more responsibilities in coordinating nursing service.

The essential responsibilities of professional nurses changed, as a result, to include the giving of skilled nursing care; health teaching and counseling; making accurate observations and communicating them to others; selecting, training, and guiding auxiliary personnel; and planning health services to meet community needs.[3] These demands on nurses required a sound and scientific nurse training to meet the challenges that the expansion of science is imposing on the profession.

In addition to the two technical programs that exist for the training of nurse assistants, two other levels of nursing education existed in Canada. The preparation of one level of practice was carried at the university level and the other in a diploma program at the post–high school level. The university program provided a sound foundation of theory and practice with an academic preparation for leadership positions in nursing.[10] Postbasic education was also available to nurses in different areas and was offered in the universities. In 1942 the University of Toronto established the first integrated basic baccalaureate program, and the University of Western Ontario in 1959 was the first to offer a course leading to a master's degree in nursing.[14,15,18]

In 1965 basic baccalaureate programs in Canada fell into two classifications—integrated and nonintegrated. The integrated program leading to a baccalaureate was conducted as an integral part of the university, whereas the nonintegrated nursing program was divided between the university that offered the science courses and the diploma school of nursing that provided the nursing portion of the program.[18] However, this trend changed in 1970, when all universities offering the nonintegrated program started to offer the integrated one.

NURSING STUDIES

The first major study of nursing in Canada was a joint effort of the Canadian Nurses' Association and the Canadian Medical Association. It was completed in 1932 by Dr. George Weir. The study, which focused on nursing and nursing education, at the time concluded that changes should be made in the system of nursing education, and it recommended removal of nursing schools from hospital control.[16]

An experimental program in nursing education was started in 1948 under the sponsorship of the Canadian Nurses' Association, the Canadian Red Cross, and the Department of National Health and Welfare. The evaluation of the project, carried over a five-year period, showed that a clinical nurse could be trained in two years. As a result, many schools of nursing reorganized their programs to include a two-year basic training period followed by a final year of internship. This became known as the "2 + 1" pattern.[16]

A 1950 study provided valuable data on the supply of nurses. It was conducted by the Committee on Public Health Practice, headed by Dr. J. H. Baillie and Lyle Creelman, a nurse who was internationally known for her extensive work with the World Health Organization. The study showed a wide range of nursing practices in the city and rural districts that did not meet individual health needs. This led to an increase in the number of schools offering public health programs and to the establishment of a university-level postbasic degree in public health.[12]

Studies, experiments, and plans are widespread in the presentday nursing profession and are increasing in popularity. Some have contributed to the solution of many problems in nursing, whereas the benefits of others are still unknown. However, these studies have aroused public interest in nursing, leading to a greater sense of responsibility on the part of the government, the people, and many members of the nursing and medical professions.

PRESENT TRENDS IN NURSING EDUCATION

In 1965 the two-year diploma program of correlated theory and practice followed by a year of internship gave way to the new two-year program. Independence from hospital control was also achieved through creation of a school management committee as the governing body for the school. Previously, diploma schools of nursing were under the direct administration of the hospital nursing departments. The responsibility of the school administration is now vested in one person, whose main interest and job is nursing education. This change has facilitated a shift from apprentice teaching to a learner-centered program, in which students utilize hospital areas to fulfill educational objectives.[13,21]

Today the student in a Canadian diploma program is taught nursing principles and their application to specific nursing situations. Content focuses on health and the factors related to the levels of wellness and the preparation of the student to meet the health needs of individuals, families, and the community. Courses are presented in broad areas related to fundamentals of nursing care, nursing in physical and mental illnesses, and maternal and child care. Pharmacology, history of nursing, ethics, legal aspects, rehabilitation, and various therapies are integrated in the major nursing areas rather than presented as separate subjects. The new curriculum stresses both prevention and cure and hence utilizes community as well as hospital facilities.[21]

Several revisions have also been introduced to the basic university course. The curriculum provides a basic professional preparation that includes qualification for the practice of hospital and public health nursing; it also qualifies nurses for teaching, administrative, and research positions. In the four-year program nursing theory and practice are integrated and associated with studies in the humanities and the sciences. Graduates are expected to show a capacity for leadership in assessing, planning, providing, and evaluating nursing care. They also receive an educational base for further study as practitioners, teachers, administrators, consultants, and researchers.[2]

Twenty-two universities in Canada offer integrated basic courses leading to the Bachelor of Science degree. The nonintegrated courses, referred to earlier, have been phased out. Many of these universities also offer baccalaureate degree courses to registered nurses who are interested in adding to and deepening their knowledge in nursing. Another development in nursing education at the university level is the introduction of postgraduate courses in nursing at the master's level to prepare nurses for leadership and research positions.[2]

EXPANDED ROLE OF THE NURSE

A joint committee of the Canadian Nurses' Association and the Canadian Medical Association met in 1972 to discuss the expanded role of the nurse. A general agreement existed among the participants that the improvement and effectiveness of Canadian health services could be better achieved by expanding the role of the nurse than by creating a new category of health workers. As a result, the nurse practitioner's role was created, which expands into many areas such as obstetrics, pediatrics, orthopedics, family care, and primary health care.[4]

This educational program for nurse practitioners originated at the University of Toronto in response to a need for additional preparation of nurses to serve the northern Canadian population. Soon after, short courses were developed in six Canadian universities to assist nurses to move into practice in primary care settings.[8] McMaster University in Hamilton, Ontario, has two undergraduate programs in the health field—one in medicine and the other in nursing. Both programs give high priority to the preparation of primary care physicians and nurses. This program was the result of an effort by educators and practitioners in nursing and medicine, with social workers making major contributions to the planning and operation of such services.[9] This program presently is offered to graduate nurses with state registration.

Teaching in the nurse practitioner program is shared by the faculties of medicine and nursing. Educational objectives cover four broad areas: assessing health needs, including history taking and physical examination; planning, which emphasizes a problem-solving approach; management of common illnesses and deviations from normal; and evaluation of the health care provided. Deviations from the pattern are common and intended to meet the diversity of student needs.[8,23] The work done by these graduates has been praised by physicians and other health workers. They support the new expanded role of the nurse and believe that nurses can be trained to practice the delivery of primary health care and hence relieve the physician for the more complicated and specialized aspects of treatment.

REFERENCES

1. Carpenter, H.: Canadian conference on nursing, Canadian Journal of Public Health **49:**34-37, 1958.
2. Carpenter, H.: The Canadian scene, International Nursing Review **21**(2): 43-48, 1974.
3. Carpenter, H.: The role of the nurse in the total health program, International Nursing Review **4:**24-30, Oct., 1957.
4. Expanded role of the nurse, Candaian Nurse **69:**23-25, 1973.
5. Gibbon, J. M., and Mathewson, M. S.: Three centuries of Canadian nursing, Toronto, 1947, The Macmillan Co.
6. Gunn, J.: Centralization of teaching in schools for nurses, Modern Hospital **16:**51-53, 1921.
7. Jensen, D. M.: History and trends of professional nursing, St. Louis, 1955, The C. V. Mosby Co.
8. Jones, P. E.: Symposium on community nursing in Canada, Nursing Clinics of North America **10:**691-698, 1975.
9. Kergin, D. J.: A Canadian educational practice in family practice nursing, International Nursing Review **22:**19-22, Feb., 1975.
10. Loyer, M. A.: Should nursing education be under the domain of hospitals? Canadian Nurse **62:**25-26, 1966.
11. McCloud, C.: District nursing in Canada, American Journal of Nursing **ii:**503, 1901-2.
12. McLure, R. E.: Education of public health nursing personnel, Canadian Journal of Public Health **57:**260-262, 1966.
13. Morgan, M. P.: Planning for curriculum changes, American Journal of Nursing **68:**554-556, 1968.
14. Mussallem, H. K.: Nursing in Canada, Nursing Times **62:**1626-1629, 1966.
15. Mussallem, H. K.: Nursing in Canada from pioneering history to a modern federation, International Nursing Review **15**(1):29-34, 1968.
16. Mussallem, H. K.: Studies on nursing in Canada, International Nursing Review **14:**35-42, June, 1967.
17. Nutting, M. A., and Dock, L. L.: A history of nursing Vol. 3, New York, 1910, G. P. Putnam's Sons.
18. Rowsell, G. S.: University nursing education—facts and trends, Canadian Nurse **62:**31-33, 1966.
19. Sellew, G., and Ebel, E.: A history of nursing, ed. 3, St. Louis, 1955, The C. V. Mosby Co.
20. Seymer, L.: A general history of nursing, London, 1935, Faber & Faber, Ltd.
21. Steed, M. E.: Trends in diploma nursing education, Canadian Nurse **64:**40-41, 1968.

22. Stewart, I., and Austin, A.: A history of nursing, New York, 1962. G. P. Putnam's Sons.
23. Wood, T.: The practice of medicine by nurses: an opinion, Canadian Medical Association Journal **114:**947, 1976.

Chapter 13

THE UNITED STATES OF AMERICA

Although nursing is as old as the human race, productive efforts to achieve professional status in the United States dates back little more than a century to the beginning of an organized system of nursing in 1873. The pioneering work done by women during the Civil War contributed to the establishment of trained nursing in the country. These women had no training as nurses but had a high degree of skill that they acquired through practice.[9]

In 1873 the first American schools that adopted the Nightingale system were established at Bellevue Hospital in New York City, at the New Haven Hospital in Connecticut, and at Massachusetts General Hospital in Boston (Fig. 7).[5] The Women's Hospital in Philadelphia and the New England Hospital for Women and Children had striven for years to train nurses.[22] In 1861 the Women's Hospital in Philadelphia opened a school that was organized and conducted by two women physicians. This attempt was unsuccessful, and the school was reorganized in 1872, to be endowed by a Dr. Dodd.[20] In addition, the New England Hospital for Women and Children, under the direction of Marie Zakrzewsky, began teaching nurses as early as 1860. Training of nurses in that school was rudimentary until Suzan Dimock took over in 1872 and reorganized the school under the Kaiserwerth system.[10] Linda Richards was the first trained nurse to graduate from this school, and later through personal contact with Miss Nightingale, she organized the New England Hospital School, with a nurse instead of a physician as head of the nursing staff.[10,17]

After the pioneer period, schools were founded at a rapid rate in many hospitals throughout the country. The Red Cross Hospital, started in New York before 1900 by Clara Barton, trained nurses for service during war and natural disasters. The course took two years and three months, and the title "Red Cross Sister" was given to graduates. The school failed grad-

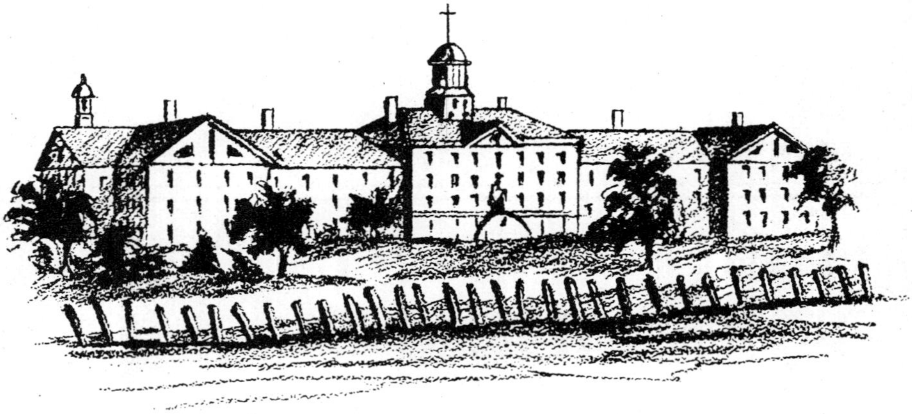

FIG. 7

Originally Bellevue Hospital was established as the New York Public Workhouse. The name was taken from its second site, Belle Vue on Kip's Farm, where it still stands. (From DeLoughery, G. L.: History and trends of professional nursing, ed. 8, St. Louis, 1977, The C. V. Mosby Co.)

ually as many of the demands for training nurses were fulfilled by the new modern schools that were developing in connection with the hospitals.[13,23] Up to this point the nursing school was a part of the hospital and was accordingly administered by a number of the medical staff.[9] Hospitals saw the schools as an economic advantage that provided better nursing care for their patients. Few, however, recognized the importance of the schools in providing skilled nurses for their community.[19]

NURSING ORGANIZATIONS

In 1879 the new graduate nurses of the New York City Hospital were urged by the Mayor of New York to form a central headquarters in the city, thus making nurses accessible to the public. As a result, the New York Agency for Trained Nurses was formed by Adelaide Mabie, which in 1886 she renamed the Philomena Society—the first organization of graduate nurses in the United States.

In the early 1890s small local groups and alumni associations began to organize and later joined together to form the basis for a national association.[13] The first steps were taken by the graduates of the Bellevue Hospital School of Nursing in 1899. They formed an alumni association whose chief purpose was to foster fellowship, mutual support, and school loyalty and to provide economic assistance in case of need.[23] Isabel Hampton was the first nurse to push the idea of a national nurses' association, as early as 1890.

In 1893, at the World's Fair in Chicago, a group of nursing leaders met to consider the development of national standards and administrative practices of schools of nursing. During the same meeting the group explored the possibilities of organizing a national nursing society. As a result of these talks, the American Society of Superintendents of Training Schools of the United States was established. The Nurses' Associated Alumni of the United States and Canada, with Isabel Hampton as president, came into existence at the same meeting and concerned itself mainly with memberships. In 1911 this same organization was named the American Nurses' Association. This historical meeting was the genesis of organized nursing in America.[9]

The purpose of the American Nurses' Association was to establish and maintain a code of ethics, to elevate the standards of nursing education and practice, to promote the usefulness and honor of the profession, and to further the financial and other interests of nurses and the profession.[13] The Society of Superintendents continued to devote its efforts to educational advancement and in 1912 changed its name to the National League of Nursing Education. This organization, by providing educational opportunities for students at the school and university levels, was a leading force for educational progress in nursing in the United States. A third organization came into being in 1912 as an expression of the growing importance of the visiting nursing or public health service. This was known as the National Organization for Public Health Nursing. Lillian Wald, the creator of the Henry Street Settlement Visiting Nurse Service and pioneer who set in motion the development of school nursing, the U.S. Children's Bureau, and the Town and County Nursing Service of the American Red Cross, was its first president.[10,21]

Sophia Palmer, one of the leading members of the National League of Nursing Education urged New York State to pass a law that would require supervision of all ot its nursing schools by the University of the State of New York and the licensing of all graduate nurses after they passed a theoretical and practical examination. During the same year Mary Davis, one of Sophia Palmer's friends, launched the first issue of the *American Journal of Nursing* under Sophia Palmer's editorship. The registration of nurses and the fight for state legislation were the main issues launched by the journal.[12,23] This impetus led to establishment of nurse registration laws in North Carolina, New Jersey, New York, and Virginia in 1903 and in the rest of the states by 1923. State registration acts brought about definite improvements and uniformity in nursing school programs, leading many schools to adopt the three-year training program that later became the standard for nursing education.[11,15]

The National League of Nursing Education Committee, with Adelaide Nutting as chairman, prepared and issued a book in 1917 on a standardized curriculum for schools of nursing, including teaching and administrative recommendations. Also, in 1912, the National Organization for Public Health Nursing established voluntary and official agencies for home and community nursing services. It also supervised and evaluated postgraduate courses in public health nursing. All national associations had many goals and interests in common, and although they performed different functions, they worked together closely for the improvement of nursing at all levels.[23]

NURSING EDUCATION

The advance of preventive medicine and public health and expansion of the nurses' field emphasized the need for a broader and sounder education than the hospital schools of the day offered. In addition, the Spanish-American War brought dissatisfaction with the haphazard trend of nursing education at the time. All these factors provided an opportunity for the American Nurses' Association to demonstrate its usefulness to the public.[15] (See Fig. 8.) The solution to the problem depended on the establishment of graduate education for those nurses who were in charge of education of nursing students in the various schools. As a result, a committee with Isabel Hampton Robb as chairman and Adelaide Nutting as a member organized a course with the help of a Dr. James S. Russell at Teachers College, Columbia University, New York. Regular courses in psychology, science, and household economics were offered to selected graduate students at the university, whereas special courses in nursing were provided at the school of nursing itself.[15] Gradually, this course expanded, and in 1907 Nutting became the first professor of nursing at the university. A new department in administration was then established that included the division of hospital economics. This department, under Nutting's guidance, gained international fame and attracted nurses from many parts of the world.[13]

Connections with the university world had a profound influence on the profession. Many liberal-minded educators became interested in problems of nursing schools and, as a result, gave invaluable advice and support to the development of the profession. The movement stimulated many changes among nurses themselves, who saw the need for a better balance between theory and practice, the science and art of nursing, and the processes of education and training. Nurses began to set their own aims and policies, define their roles, and study their problems more objectively in the light of fundamental principles and the wide experience of various education experts.[23]

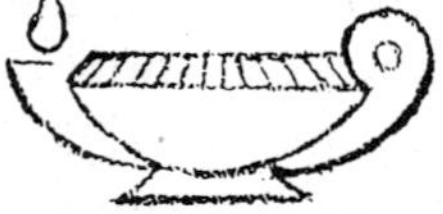

FIG. 8

Nursing education lamp. (From DeLoughery, G. L.: History and trends of professional nursing, ed. 8, St. Louis, 1977, The C. V. Mosby Co.)

At the basic education level a preparatory course was developed by Nutting at the Johns Hopkins Hospital in 1901, but it received little support.[6] However, in 1909 a full course in nursing was established at the University of Minnesota by Dr. Richard Beard, under the direction of Louise Powell. This course was the pioneer in basic nursing education at the university level.[10,23] The University of Cincinnati and Teachers College offered courses in nursing education in 1916 in a program that led to a degree. In 1923 the first independent university school was established at Yale University, with its own dean and a substantial endowment by Annie Goodrich.[10] Students in this program completed two years of college work before entering the hospital for an additional twenty-eight months of experience, at the end of which a bachelor's degree in nursing was granted.[6] Gradually nursing, like many other professions, found a permanent place in many United States universities that were flexible in combing academic and professional studies.

Two developments of nursing education were the gradual improvement in entrance requirements and the introduction of a preliminary course preceding the graduate course. In addition, special training was required of visiting nurse trainees, resulting in the development of a postgraduate course in public health nursing at New York City Teachers College. After 1914 public health nursing was gradually becoming an integral part of all higher education curricula in all the professional schools of nursing.[13,23]

Meanwhile, to help meet long-term demand for military nurses, the army school of nursing was organized in 1918 during World War I, with Annie Goodrich as dean. A three-year course with a special nine months' credit to college graduates constituted the curriculum.[15] The American Red Cross and Vassar College also offered a three-month preliminary course to college graduates, some of whom were nursing graduates. In civilian hospitals and homes the war created a real shortage of nurses. This resulted in the development of a health education course that was offered to housewives and conducted by well-trained nurses. Although this plan, organized by Jane Delano, was opposed by many nurse educators of the day, the American Red Cross has continued to offer these courses as an important peacetime activity.[13,15] Another consequence of the war was the establishment of nursing military status achieved through the diligent efforts of many nurses who served during the war. Julia Stimson, then Superintendent of the Army Nurse Corps, received the rank of major, and other army nurses were given corresponding ranks.

The war also highlighted the need for more developments in medical and health-related fields. Several studies were initiated by nurses and supported by the Rockefeller Foundation and other agencies, the outcome of which strengthened the position of nurses and brought about the combination of health teaching with nursing service. An immediate result of one study was the establishment of an experimental demonstration school at Yale University, endowed by the Rockefeller Foundation, and a similar one at Western Reserve University, endowed by Francis Balton.

NURSING STUDIES

After the publication of the Winslow-Goldmark report, the Committee on the Grading of Nursing Schools was formed in 1926, with representatives from medical, nursing, and hospital organizations. The purpose of this committee was to help raise the standards of nursing schools by means of a classification system to make it possible to give recognition to those schools of good standing and to stimulate others to improve their standards. A five-year program was adopted in 1926 to cover projects such as the supply and demand for nursing service, job analysis of nursing and nurse teaching, and actual grading of nursing schools. The practical results of this study were the elimination of inferior schools and the requirement of a high school degree for admission to all schools of nursing in the country. It also led to the accrediting of nursing schools by the National League of Nursing Education, which set the standards for general evaluation. It was the responsibility of every school to apply to the committee for accreditation. The committee, in turn, had to judge the services and publish a list that would contain all schools that had satisfactorily met the criteria set by the committee.[13,23]

THE ASSOCIATION OF COLLEGIATE SCHOOLS OF NURSING

The Association of Collegiate Schools of Nursing was established in 1933 and was composed of basic and postgraduate schools of nursing that were of a collegiate type and that formed a part of an accredited college or university. The association was unique in the sense that members aimed at the improvement of their programs through their own activities and not through outside accrediting agencies.[12] The objectives and aims of the group included the development of nursing education on a professional and collegiate level, the promotion and strengthening of relations between nursing and institutions of higher education, and the promotion of study and experimentation in nursing service and nursing education. Emphasis was placed on reducing the lag between curriculum development through nursing research. The Association of Collegiate Schools of Nursing brought its plans to fruition by developing the periodical, *Nursing Research,* in 1952. Annie Goodrich was the first president of this association.

THE BROWN REPORT

The National Nursing Council for War Service was organized in 1940 by the three national associations, and representatives from the American Red Cross and the nursing agencies of the federal government. This association proved to be an effective link between organized nursing schools and the federal government and supplied an adequate number of nurses to serve the Armed Forces during World War II. Toward the end of the war, *The Brown Report* on Nursing for the Future was published. Dr. Esther Lucille Brown, Director of the Department of Studies in Professions of the Russell Sage Foundation, served as director of the study that resulted in the report. The report stressed that the term "professional" in nursing should be used only for those who have studied in a school accredited by the National League for Nursing. Education and legislation for the training of practical nurses was recommended. The report also emphasized that all nursing schools should be nationally classified and accredited, that collegiate faculty standards should be accepted in all schools, and that a school of nursing should be affiliated with a university and should have a separate budget.[13,23]

AUXILIARY NURSING

Meanwhile, practical preparation and licensing were being actively promoted by the National Association for Practical Nurse Education, formed during the war under the leadership of Hilda Torrop. In 1949 the National Federation of Licensed Practical Nurses was organized to bring together all practical nurses who met the standards. Gradually, the professional nurses' organizations came to accept this new branch in nursing and helped to establish its standards and prepare students joining it. Programs for the training of nurses' aides became more popular and gained more acceptance among nurses. As a result, nurses' aides began to perform many of the errands that nurses had previously done and even performed some of the less technical nursing procedures. Many of these nurses' aides eventually became practical nurses when licensing for practical nurses was instituted.[23]

ASSOCIATE DEGREE NURSING

Experiments in nursing education conducted by representatives of junior colleges and of nursing educators followed later. This movement was intended to try out a combined academic and technical curriculum qualifying graduates for state registration as nurses. Teachers College, Columbia University, took the initiative in planning and conducting such programs under the direction of Louise McManus and Mildred Montag. Community college programs in nursing followed publication of Mildred

Montag's doctoral thesis, *Education of Nursing Technicians,* written in 1951.[13] The associate degree program, which is widespread in the United States, offers a two-year curriculum in technical nursing. When this program is viewed from the historical vantage point, it appears to have contributed as a catalytic agent to the nursing profession in its identification of levels of preparation for nursing practice.[8]

RESTRUCTURING NURSING ASSOCIATIONS

As a result of rapid developments in nursing education, all the nursing associations, which included the National League of Nursing Education, the American Nurses' Association, the National Organization for Public Health Nurses, the National Association for Colored Graduate Nurses, the Association of Collegiate Schools of Nursing, and the American Association of Industrial Nurses decided to merge into two organizations. One, a somewhat reorganized American Nurses' Association, was composed entirely of nurses and spoke entirely for the profession. The other, the National League for Nursing, which included nurses and non-nurses, individual and corporate members, represented all those responsible for the sound development and support of nursing services and nursing schools.[23]

The American College of Nurse-Midwifery, organized in 1955, has been highly regarded as an instigator of legislation and certification requirements and as a source of guidelines for nurse-midwives in the United States. *The Bulletin of the American College of Nurse-Midwifery* is its official publication.

MALE NURSES

Trained professional male nurses functioned in the United States as early as 1910. According to the United States census of that year, approximately 7% of all student and graduate nurses were men. However, the percentage declined to 2% in 1940. Most male nurses at that time were graduates of hospital schools of nursing connected with psychiatric institutions. Although male nurses were included in the American Nurses' Association, no special attention was given to them before the formation of the Men Nurses' Section of the American Nurses' Association in 1940.[6] Men in the nursing field obviously have suffered from the same discrimination that women have experienced in other fields. For instance, in World War II, when nurses had gained relative rank first and then regular rank, male nurses were kept in enlisted grades. This discrimination was not the responsibility of female nurses themselves, since in 1902 the law organizing the Army Nurse Corps defined nurses as females and so did the law that established the Navy Nurse Corps in 1908.[6]

The changing status of the male nurse was finally recognized by the United States army in 1954. Also, the growing need for male nurses in the

Veterans Administration Hospitals, in the psychiatric hospitals, and in general hospitals made it easier for male nurses to find employment. Many schools of nursing started recruiting male students, and positions in public health, sanitation, and administration were made available.[6] Also, opportunities in the fields of anesthesia and occupational health made them more interesting to prospective male students.[15]

At present, male nurses are found in almost all nursing fields; they have assumed leadership positions in national nursing organizations by serving on the American Nurses' Association Board of Directors and on the National League for Nursing staff.[15] In the future, employment of greater numbers of male nurses may contribute to solving the worldwide shortage of nurses. (See Fig. 9.)

Along the same line, and as evidenced repeatedly throughout history, the struggle of nursing to be a profession has been an integral part of women's movements. Few male nurses took leading roles in the development of nursing in earlier days. Hence, this development has always paralleled influences affecting women's status. As a result, nursing was predominantly seen and referred to as a woman's profession. Undoubtedly,

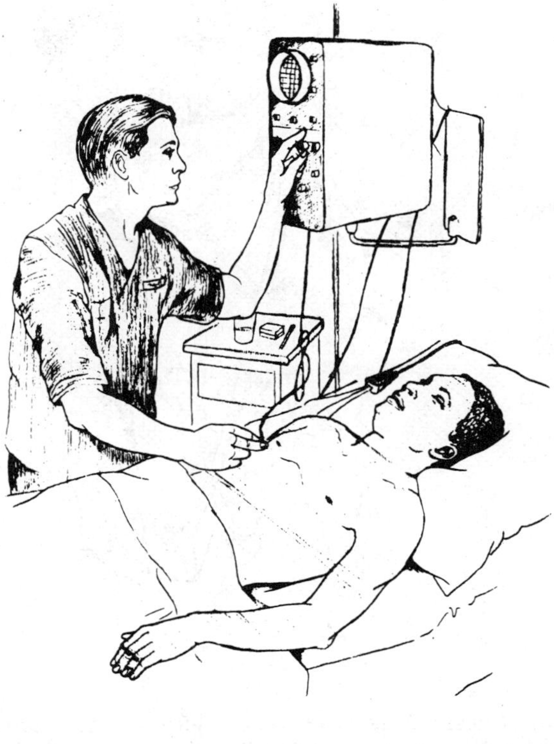

FIG. 9

Nursing is becoming an increasingly popular occupation for men as it expands in scope, especially in the associate degree programs. (From DeLoughery, G. L.: History and trends of professional nursing, ed. 8, St. Louis, 1977, The C. V. Mosby Co.)

nursing has provided women with an early opportunity to express themselves and to acquire education.[3] At present the profession is challenged to keep abreast with other professions while working for the general interest of both men and women.

NURSING SERVICES

With increasing demands on nursing services during the 1960s, specialization in different nursing fields gained popularity. Many more nurses were needed in clinical specialties such as medical-surgical nursing, maternal and child nursing, psychiatric nursing, rehabilitative nursing, and community and public health nursing. Other specialized areas include the military, government health field research, the Peace Corps, and international organizations such as the World Health Organization.[13] These specialty areas expand the field of nursing from simple nursing situations to complex care requiring a better trained nurse.[2]

The development of the nurse clinician and the clinical nurse spe-

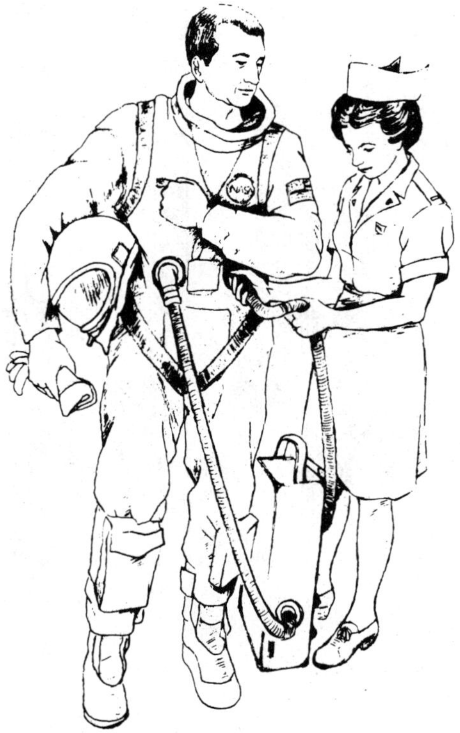

FIG. 10

One of the most exciting fields in modern life, the space program, presents new opportunities for the nurse's special skills. (From DeLoughery, G. L.: History and trends of professional nursing, ed. 8, St. Louis, 1977, The C. V. Mosby Co.)

cialist was a response to the growing need for more specialized nurses. This evolving role requires postgraduate educational preparation presently offered at the master's level or beyond.[13] Subspecialty areas are also available for nurses interested in focusing on a specific branch of nursing, such as cardiac nursing. There is increasing demand in the field of nurse-midwifery. The first nurse-midwifery school in the United States was opened in 1935, and ever since many universities have offered courses on the graduate level, resulting from a growing need for better antepartum and obstetrical care for mothers and newborns.[7]

.In addition to the foregoing, the Army Nurse Corps, the Navy Nurse Corps, the Air Force Nurse Corps and aerospace nursing were established as a result of the dynamic changes in society, requiring fundamental changes in the nursing profession (Fig. 10). The very nature of nursing, as well as the range of functions from basic to specialized nursing tasks that the profession can offer, have resulted in the need for more than one kind of nurse. Beside the variety of challenging services that these nursing branches offer, their job security has proved to be attractive to nurses. Personnel policies; complete hospital, medical, surgical, and dental care; health services to dependents; and continuous pay increases for all grades are some of the benefits that accompany these positions in the services.[13]

THE PEACE CORPS

The Peace Corps came into being in 1961 with the objective of promoting world peace and friendship. Registered nurses were recruited from all levels to serve as volunteers or as Peace Corps nurses. This again has opened a wide door for nurses interested in helping people and in promoting worldwide friendship.[13] United States nurses work side by side with nurses of host countries in hospitals, rural clinics, and health centers. Other nurses assist with the clinical teaching of nursing students or auxiliary personnel. The Peace Corps has proved to be effective in promoting a better understanding by United States citizens of other people's cultures and beliefs.[15]

NURSING TRENDS

In a dynamic society and a period of rapid change, strain is imposed on institutions and professions. No longer is the old method of educating nurses adequate to meet the demands of society. As a result, the role of registered nurses is expanding significantly as nurses take more responsibility for diagnosing and treating patients. This has begun to create a significant realignment of health care roles because traditionally physicians have been considered the only diagnostic and treatment decision makers. Factors that influence this trend have been attributed to the women's movement and to the progress in medical science and technology that have expanded the range of services a physician can perform. Advancement in science has also stimulated interest in specialization to the extent that, at present, specialists outnumber general practitioners. This trend creates a shortage of physicians who are available for first level, or primary, care.[4]

The gap created by the physician in the health care delivery system is presently filled by the physician's assistant and the nurse practitioner. The first program to train physician's assistants was started at Duke University in 1965 to prepare excorpsmen in two years to perform the less complex medical tasks. In the United States at present fifty accredited programs train physician's assistants, who are allowed to practice in thirty-seven states.[4] However, as early as 1962 public health nurses functioning as nurse practitioners in North Carolina and elsewhere in the country were giving primary care in informal situations.

The role of the nurse practitioner is described as the expanded role of the nurse and is rapidly developing to meet the needs of the health care system. A Nurse Training Act was passed in 1971 authorizing nurses with special preparation to diagnose and treat patients.[4] At the beginning nursing schools were reluctant to include diagnostic content in their curricula, and nurses were worried about the safety and morality of violating laws. Now the barrier is being slowly removed, and many states have revised or are in the process of revising their laws, breaking down the traditions and developing a momentum for change.

Nurse practitioners are now licensed to carry their own practice and be accountable to their own clients for maintaining standards of practice. Primary care provided at a satellite facility in a rural or urban area or in acute care settings, such as intensive care units where there is a need for prompt decisions from the nurse, is available and represents settings where nurses can work in their expanded role.[1]

The American Nurses' Association has defined the term "practitioner" to mean an individual who has completed a program of study leading to competence as a registered nurse in an expanded role whose duty and responsibility encompass, for example, obtaining a health history, assessing health illness status, entering a person into the health care system, sustaining and supporting during diagnosis and therapy persons who are impaired or ill, managing a care regimen for acute and chronically ill patients, counseling, and supervision.[1] In other words the nurse practitioner is presently well on the way to becoming a major health provider of the future who will be the gatekeeper to the health care delivery system. Health maintenance and prevention will be the key functions of the nurse practitioner.[14] A general agreement exists among nurse educators that the preparation of these nurses should be at the graduate level and that the graduate program should be improved to include all aspects for the training of nurses in the expanded role.[14]

As a result of the explosion of knowledge and the development of new techniques in medicine and health care, continuing education for the health worker is being mandated. It is only through ongoing education that the gap between knowledge explosion in health care and the delivery of improved health care services can be closed. The knowledge explosion has required many professionals and practitioners to show proof of competence and to keep their knowledge and skills up to date.[18]

In nursing the first National Conference for Directors of Continuing Education was approved by the American Nurses' Association Commission on Education in 1971.[16] In 1974 the American Nurses' Association stated its support and assistance in the development of state systems for the institution of mandatory continuing education. California was the first state to pass legislation laws providing continuing education requirements for registered nurses. Licenses can only be renewed on submission of proof of participation in education courses. This law took effect in July, 1978.[16] Many other states are establishing similar laws.

The ladder concept, or the open curriculum, in nursing is another trend that allows for career mobility in the profession. Many colleges give blanket credits to diploma and associate degree graduates with the promise of a bachelor of science degree on completion of some upper division courses covering an average period of one and one-half years. This resulted from the strong stand of the Regents External Degree of the University of the State of New York that nursing at the university level should be a right of everyone and that those who could not attend a college but acquired knowledge and skills through other sources should not be denied the recognition to which they were entitled.[13] This concept is gaining acceptance and has been adopted by colleges of nursing in several parts of the United States.

Another trend in nursing education is the specialization of nurses at the doctoral level. Graduates of doctoral programs in nursing engage in consultation, research, teaching, or the administration of nursing service. However, they would always be high-level clinical practitioners, for example, nurse teachers who remain involved in clinical practice while teaching.

NURSING RESEARCH

Scientific knowledge coupled with scientific inquiry is the keystone to professionalism and further growth of any profession. Any new knowledge added to a profession is introduced through research, and research in nursing is expanding rapidly. Results of such progress have shown tremendous effects on the administration of patient care and will likely be a determining factor in revolutionizing the health care delivery system in the United States. In the not too distant past, much research was devoted to the improvement of nursing education and not to nursing service. However, with the expanded role of nurses and the new responsibilities that nurses are carrying in the hospital and community, this trend is rapidly changing and much current research focuses on developments in nursing care and the improvement of the health care delivery system.

This impact on research was reinforced in 1955 by the establishment of the American Nurses' Foundation for organized research in nursing and patient care, which was endorsed by the American Nurses' Association. The foundation publishes *Directory of Nurses Holding Earned Doctorates* and funds small grants to support nursing research. Another organization, the Council of Nurse Researchers comprises nurses with master's or higher nursing degrees who are engaged in conducting research or in guiding nursing students or registered nurses in research. Functions of the council include exchange of research findings at conventions, institutes, and other meetings of the American Nurses' Association. In addition to facilitating research both within the profession and in collaboration with other disciplines, the council provides recognition of excellence and achievement in the field or nursing research.

REFERENCES

1. Abdellah, F.: Nursing practitioners and nursing practice, American Journal of Public Health **66:**245-246, 1976.
2. American Nurses' Association first position on education for nursing, American Journal of Nursing **65:**106-111, 1965.
3. Brand, K. L.: Perils and parallels of women in nursing, Nursing Forum **14:** 160-174, 1975.
4. Bullough, B.: Influence on role expansion, American Journal of Nursing **76:** 1476-1481, 1976.
5. Bullough, V.: The origin of modern American nursing, Nursing Forum **2:**13, 1963.
6. Bullough, V., and Bullough, B.: The emergence of modern nursing, ed. 2, London, 1969, The Macmillan Co.
7. Day, P. E.: A symposium on nursing in America: nursing history in the states, Nursing Mirror **143:**45-48, July 8, 1976.
8. Dechow, G. H.: Associate degree nursing education, Journal of Nursing Education **5:**3-4, 1966.
9. Dietz, L. D.: History and modern nursing, Philadelphia, 1963, F. A. Davis Co.
10. Dock, L., and Stewart, M.: A short history of nursing, New York, 1938, G. P. Putnam's Sons.
11. Dolan, J.: Goodnow's history of nursing, Philadelphia, 1958, W. B. Saunders Co.
12. Frank, Sister M. C.: The historical development of nursing, Philadelphia, 1953, W. B. Saunders Co.
13. Griffin, G., and Griffin, J.: History and trends of professional nursing, St. Louis, 1973, The C. V. Mosby Co.
14. Haase, P. T.: Pathways for practice, American Journal of Nursing **76:**950-954, 1976.
15. Jameison, E., Sewall, M., and Suhrie, E.: Trends in nursing history, ed. 6, Philadelphia, 1966, W. B. Saunders Co.

16. Kuramoto, A. B.: Professional education and its implications for continuing education, Journal of Continuing Education for Nurses **6:**8-11, 1975.
17. Nutting, M. A., and Dock, L. L.: A history of nursing, New York, 1907, G. P. Putnam's Sons.
18. Peplau, H. E.: What future for nursing? AORN Journal **24:**217-235, 1976.
19. Rogers, C.: The birth of our profession, AORN Journal **11:**73, 1970.
20. Sellew, G., and Ebel, E.: A history of nursing, St. Louis, 1955, The C. V. Mosby Co.
21. Seymer, L. R.: A general history of nursing, London, 1932, Faber & Faber Ltd.
22. Shryock, R.: The history of nursing, Philadelphia, 1959, W. B. Saunders Co.
23. Stewart, I., and Austin, A.: A history of nursing, New York, 1962, G. P. Putnam's Sons.

Chapter 14

LATIN AMERICA

Spanish and Portuguese religious orders were responsible for early nursing in Latin America. The Sisters trained women of the upper-servant class for hospital and private duty nursing. Practical teaching was mainly done in the convents, after which the women were sent to various private or city hospitals to learn there by practice under physicians. The only educational requirement was that trainees should know how to read and write. However, when European and American residents emigrated to South America, they established private hospitals and nursing homes to care for their own people. Also, mission hospitals established in South America had an influence on the foundation of modern nursing. Moreoever, the development of better nursing care was due to the support of the medical profession and public health officials who had been in contact with modern developments in other countries. Their efforts were accompanied by attempts by the Red Cross societies to assist in establishing schools of nursing and in helping other institutions, under government auspices, to recognize nursing as a profession.[7,14]

Traditionally, young women in the Spanish and Portuguese cultures have seldom left the house to enter professions, since they are expected to remain at home until they were married. This permitted the influx of foreign nurses, especially from Britain, who introduced the Nightingale system and organized schools of nursing similar to that of St. Thomas's Hospital in London. As early as 1912, Dr. Carlos Nery, acting for the Department of Charities, brought several English nurses to Montevideo, Uruguay, to start a nursing school modeled after the Nightingale system. The English nurses remained for three years, leaving their first graduates to take over what they had started.[7,12]

However, because of middle class prohibitions against working women and a resistance of the middle and upper class to recognize the importance of any sort of manual labor, modern nursing was slow to develop in Latin America. After Uruguay, Brazil was the first country to establish a school of nursing based on the Nightingale system. This resulted in establishment of the Anna Nery School of Nursing, founded by North American nurses in Rio de Janeiro in 1923. This school was soon run by the Brazilian nurses and in 1943 became part of the University of Brazil. Training covered a three-year period, at the end of which students were sent by the Rockefeller Foundation to the United States for further study.[3,24]

Other attempts to establish schools of nursing were made in Peru, Argentina, Ecuador, and Chile. The governments in some of these countries took the initiative in opening schools of nursing and in encouraging students to apply by making available financial aid that included scholarships to prospective students. The emphasis of these schools, however, was on public health instruction. Red Cross societies were also active in those countries in establishing schools of nursing that required three years of full-time training. Auxiliary nursing was the most widespread activity of the Red Cross schools of nursing, which were organized to meet emergencies, administer first-aid treatments, assist nurses in hospitals, or staff outpatient clinics. In the majority of cases, auxiliary nursing was performed by women of good social standing who worked primarily as volunteers to satisfy a desire for service.[10]

In 1940 the Rockefeller Foundation, the Kellogg Foundation, the Institute of Inter-American Affairs, and the Pan American Sanitary Bureau, which later became the regional office of the World Health Organization, contributed to the development of schools of nursing in Latin America. A few of the schools were similar to those in the United States, whereas others were mainly technical in emphasis. Excluding the few private and Red Cross schools of nursing, Latin American governments assumed full control over most of the nursing schools that existed at the time. Nursing laws in Bolivia, Chile, Ecuador, Peru, Uruguay, and Venezuela were enacted in the 1940s that defined the title "nurse" and laid down conditions for training. Public health nursing was also developed under the auspices of the government, and it greatly increased in demand because of its obvious need. Many short courses of four to eight months were given to graduate nurses who were interested in becoming visiting nurses.[8,14,25]

From its beginning, nursing education followed the curricula and regulations set by the government. Many schools were located in universities, but generally they did not enjoy the status of other professional schools in the same university. Schools of nursing in Brazil and Chile were exceptions, since their candidates had the same educational requirements as candidates to the school of medicine. Also, these schools integrated the teaching of social and health concepts in the basic curriculum and furnished the leadership for nursing in the Spanish-speaking world. As a result, many fellowship students from different countries joined these schools rather than going to the United States, as was the trend before 1940. The reasons for this influx, beside the progress in nursing education, were the common language and the similarity in health conditions.[4]

As suggested earlier, public health programs steadily increased in number in most Latin American countries. The cooperation of the United States in these programs contributed to the establishment of more centers, mainly in areas where no previous public health work existed. Nursing educators in these programs had been influential in persuading local nurses to seek public health nursing preparation and in developing university-based public health schools of nursing. Many of these nurses had struggled hard to establish this service and, in the process, broke many traditions; hence they paved the way for entry to the profession for many young women whose culture restricted their desire to become nurses or to do any kind of work outside the home.[18]

Through the Institute of the Inter-American Affairs, cooperative health programs of the United States and Latin America have developed since 1942. These programs included physicians, sanitary engineers, nurses, and other health workers who contributed to the transmission of influence across the border from the United States. Experts from different fields have cooperated with natives in local Latin American communities to establish programs in various health areas that were later adopted by the individual countries. Such programs emphasized the prevention of disease through health teaching and effective treatment and care. Schools of nursing consequently adopted this approach, and prevention of disease became an integral part of the curriculum. Inter-American seminars and workshops were conducted, and the World Health Organization awarded scholarships and fellowships to native candidates who had the potential to contribute to the social welfare.[3,12]

Since it is impossible to consider Latin America as a homogeneous whole, it is also difficult to speak of nursing in Latin America in simple terms. As a profession, nursing is only fifty to sixty years old in some countries, whereas in others it has been introduced recently. Because of these variations, the role the profession has played in *some* Latin American countries should be studied in the hope that this will provide a better view of some nursing practices in Central and South America. A study of the specific national settings will reflect the progress of the nursing profession in Latin America.

Brazil

Religious Roman Catholic sisterhoods were nominally the source of supply of nurses in Brazil. Nursing was done, however, by uninterested persons, men and women, who frequently were patients themselves and who showed interest in their fellow patients.[6,11] In 1921 physicians in the National Department of Health first became conscious of a need for trained nurses. As a result, Dr. Carlos Chagas visited the United States and requested the cooperation and assistance of the International Health Board. To adapt the North American system to the needs of Brazil, a Service of Nursing was established in the National Department of Health with rank equal to that of the other bureaus of the department. Brazil was the first country in the world to establish such a bureau in the National Department of Health.[19]

DEVELOPMENT OF SCHOOLS OF NURSING

Under the direction of this service, schools of nursing were established as annexes to the hospitals. Only students whose personal qualifications were of the highest order and who had a normal school diploma were accepted. The course covered a period of two years and four months and included theoretical as well as practical work. One of the first schools to be started was the Anna Nery School of Nursing, founded in 1923.[28] To provide students with a well-rounded experience in theory and practice, the length of the nursing course was extended in 1928 to three years. With the help of the Rockefeller Foundation, many graduates of this school were sent to the United States to be prepared as leaders of the profession. These graduates later replaced staff from the United States in operating the schools of nursing.

By 1925 graduates of the school felt the need for organization to further the development of the profession. This resulted in the formation of the National Association of Brazilian Graduate Nurses, which was granted membership in the International Council of Nurses in 1929 and for the first time became a part of the world nursing service. Its journal is called the *Revista Brasiliera de Enfermagen.*[25]

A decree regulating the profession of nursing was signed in 1931 by a Dr. Vargas, then chief of the provisional government of Brazil. As a result, the title of "graduate nurse" was given only to graduates holding diplomas from official schools recognized by law. The direction of the school of nursing was placed under Rachel Haddock Lobo, a nurse who had taken a postgraduate course in the United States and had experience in administration and instruction in Brazil. This step was a victory that the nursing profession had long struggled to achieve.[22]

NURSING AT THE UNIVERSITY LEVEL

Ten years after the Anna Nery School was opened, Dr. Carlos Chagas inaugurated the second school of nursing, Escola Carlos Chagas, founded on the same pattern as the Anna Nery School. For that decade the National

Association of Brazilian Graduate Nurses had struggled to place the school in the university, and by 1934 another decree was issued by the government authorizing the organization of a School of Hygiene and Public Health within the university and placing the Anna Nery School within it.[22] In 1942 the Anna Nery School of Nursing became an independent university school.[5]

The gradually changing concept of nursing functions and the entrance of well-educated young women from families of high social standing into the profession exerted a great deal of influence on the status of the profession.[1] The requirement of university-level entrance examinations for those entering the school of nursing had a significant effect in changing the profession's social status. In addition, hospitals and administrators at the public and private sectors, recognizing the difference in the quality of nursing care given by trained as opposed to untrained nurses, raised nurses' salaries—another factor that made nursing more appealing to many educated young women.[5,21]

NURSING EDUCATION

In 1949 a federal law was enacted that established two levels of nursing education: a basic three-year program requiring secondary education for admission and an eighteen-month program for practical nurses for which only practical training was required. This law also provided for accreditation of both schools of nursing and assured their funding.[5] An integrated national system was later adopted that included courses at three levels. The highest level of professional nursing schools (that is, university schools), with a four-year curriculum and regular university entrance requirements, prepared nurses for leadership and teaching positions. At the middle level the technical nursing schools prepared diploma nurses. The auxiliary schools constituted the lowest level. The government in its plan assured the progress of the individual from one level to the other through additional preparation.[9]

Postbasic and postgraduate programs in nursing education are presently available in different areas of nursing specialization, such as nursing education for those interested in becoming teachers, nursing school administrators, nursing service administrators, and public health nurses. All these specializations are acquired within a nine-month period at a specialized institution. The nurse-midwifery diploma is also available at the postgraduate level and requires one year of work in public health, obstetrical and pediatric nursing, and social welfare.[20] This progress in nursing as a profession has given the nurse a highly positive image, according to a recent Brazilian survey. Nursing students in the country attribute to the nurse the duties, aspirations, and values that reflect a high degree of commitment and dedication to the profession.[7]

Colombia

DEVELOPMENT OF SCHOOLS OF NURSING

As early as 1857, many hospitals were founded in the different parts of the country by French Sisters, who settled in Colombia at the time. This movement was later followed by other religious orders, the most influential of which was the Order of St. Vincent de Paul. In 1903 Dr. Jorge Calvo, on his return from a visit to Europe, founded the first school of nursing in Catagina. His admiration of the nursing system there inspired him to establish the school of nursing at St. Clara Hospital. In 1913 Professor José Ignacio Barberi, founder of the Children's Hospital, established another school of nursing.[13]

The first semiofficial organization for the education of nurses was established in 1924. As a result, a school of nursing was founded in Bogotá in collaboration with the faculty of medicine. The program offered by the new school integrated theory and practice, lasted for two years, and required primary education for admission. This school closed in 1937.[13]

The Red Cross in Colombia took the initiative in 1919 by importing a Belgian nurse, a Madame Ledu, who implemented modern nursing in Colombia and recruited women of a higher socioeconomic class to join the profession. In 1929 the National School of Nursing was founded with the help of the Rockefeller Foundation and contributions of North American nurses. Professor José Maria Montoya was assigned by the Colombian government to head the newly founded school. The National School of Nursing offered two programs: One prepared nurses for staff nursing positions, and the other prepared nurses for health and social assistance work throughout the country.[13]

The Red Cross of Colombia established another school in 1938 to prepare nurses for administrative positions in hospitals and clinics. The Red Cross school was the first in the country to accept student residents, opening the way for many interested nursing candidates from different parts of the country. The program adopted the American Red Cross principles in preparing nurses to work in wars and natural disasters. Thus nurses had their practical experience in military hospitals while their theoretical preparation stressed military health, orthopedics, kinesitherapy, and legal medicine.[13]

With World War II the United States government cooperated with the governments of America to expand the principles of world health by fighting infectious diseases. As a result, the Inter-American service of Public Health established a college of nutrition and a normal superior school of nursing, which were incorporated in the *Universidad Nacional* in 1943. The school of nursing was under the direction of Helen Wjouit, a North American nurse. The school was sustained by the governments of Colombia and the United States, the Rockefeller Foundation, and the *Officina Sanitaria Panamericana,* or *Pan American Sanitary Bureau*. The program was based on that of the North American schools of nursing.[13]

NURSING EDUCATION

Professional nurses and auxiliary personnel are responsible for giving nursing care in Colombia. As early as 1903, university schools of nursing provided basic nursing education. At present admission requirements to all schools of nursing are consolidated and include completion of high school. The academic university system was adopted in 1963, placing nursing students on the same level as students in other faculties. The four-year program now culminated in the degree of Licenciatura in Nursing Sciences, focusing on the natural and social sciences and the humanities and integrating nursing theory with practice. This is in contrast to nursing education in the past, which stressed the development of skills and bedside care.[23]

Continuing education in psychiatry, administration of nursing service, and public health have been developed by the National University of Colombia. Specialization in maternal-child health, psychiatric, and medical-surgical nursing is available at the master's level in most university schools of nursing. Since all the courses are offered in Spanish, which is needed for administrative and teaching positions, the nursing shortage has decreased greatly in Colombia as well as in other Latin American countries. For economic and language reasons Colombian nurses are taking advantage of these studies that they cannot obtain in other countries.[23]

The development of nursing in Colombia has been aided all along by motivated members of the profession, various international organizations such as the World Health Organization, the Kellogg Foundation, the Agency for International Development, and the Rockefeller Foundation.

BASIC NURSING EDUCATION

All schools of nursing in Colombia are approved and controlled by the Ministry of Education through the Colombian Institute for the Improvement of Higher Education. This institute is responsible for accreditation of schools of nursing, the revision of curricula, and the implementation of nursing education policies. On the other hand, the Ministries of Health and Education cooperate in administering the schools of practical nursing.[15] However, since 1969 the National Association of University Schools of Nursing has been operated as the consultant agency to the Ministry of Health. It has developed many activities toward maintaining the quality of nursing curricula and instruction. Within the university setting the schools of nursing function as autonomous units, with the main responsibility assumed by a nurse administrator.[15]

NURSING PROGRAMS

Nursing education in Colombia is on two levels: the professional and the auxiliary. Professional nursing is taught in three programs in the university: (1) postgraduate or magister, (2) Licenciatura, or the Bachelor of Science in Nursing (B.S.N.), and (3) general nursing. Auxiliary nursing, on the other hand, takes place in independent schools, schools annexed to hospitals, sectional health services, or vocational educational institutes. Auxiliary or subprofessional nursing has three divisions: (1) practical nursing, (2) aides in nursing, and (3) health promoters.[15]

Graduate programs offer master's degrees in maternal and child nursing, mental health and psychiatric nursing, medical and surgical nursing, public health nursing, administration and nursing education, and administration and nursing services. Also, short courses in community nursing, maternal and child nursing, psychiatric nursing, midwifery, and epidemiology are offered at the graduate level.[15] The Licenciatura, or B.S.N., program is four years (eight academic semesters) and is offered in nine universities throughout the country. The general nursing program, equivalent to the diploma program in the United States, requires three years (six academic semesters) of study. Contrary to the trend in the United States, the diploma program in Colombia has been flourishing—a measure attributed to the need for more nurses in this Latin American country.[15]

Thirty-two schools for auxiliary nursing presently function in Colombia. The practical nursing program requires eighteen months of study, including six months of on-the-job practice. Nurses' aides are prepared in hospitals during a three-month period according to the institution's needs. The health promoters, or *Promotoras de Salud,* are agents who are prepared through a three-month program to give primary care in rural communities.[15]

Candidates for the university nursing program should have five years of primary and six years of secondary education and must pass university entrance examinations to be accepted. Candidates for the practical nursing programs must finish two to four years of secondary education and pass the entrance examination and interview. Nursing aides are also required to have completed two years of secondary education. The *Promotoras* are recruited from their own communities. Interest in working with their own people, a minimum of five years of elementary education, and the ability to pass the entrance examination are requirements for admission to the programs. No age limit is set for the candidates to the professional programs. However, 18 years is the minimum age recommended for auxiliary personnel. Students in the auxiliary nursing programs pay no tuition fees, whereas students in the professional programs pay tuition according to scales established at the respective universities in the country.[15]

No unified curriculum for university nursing programs exists in Colom-

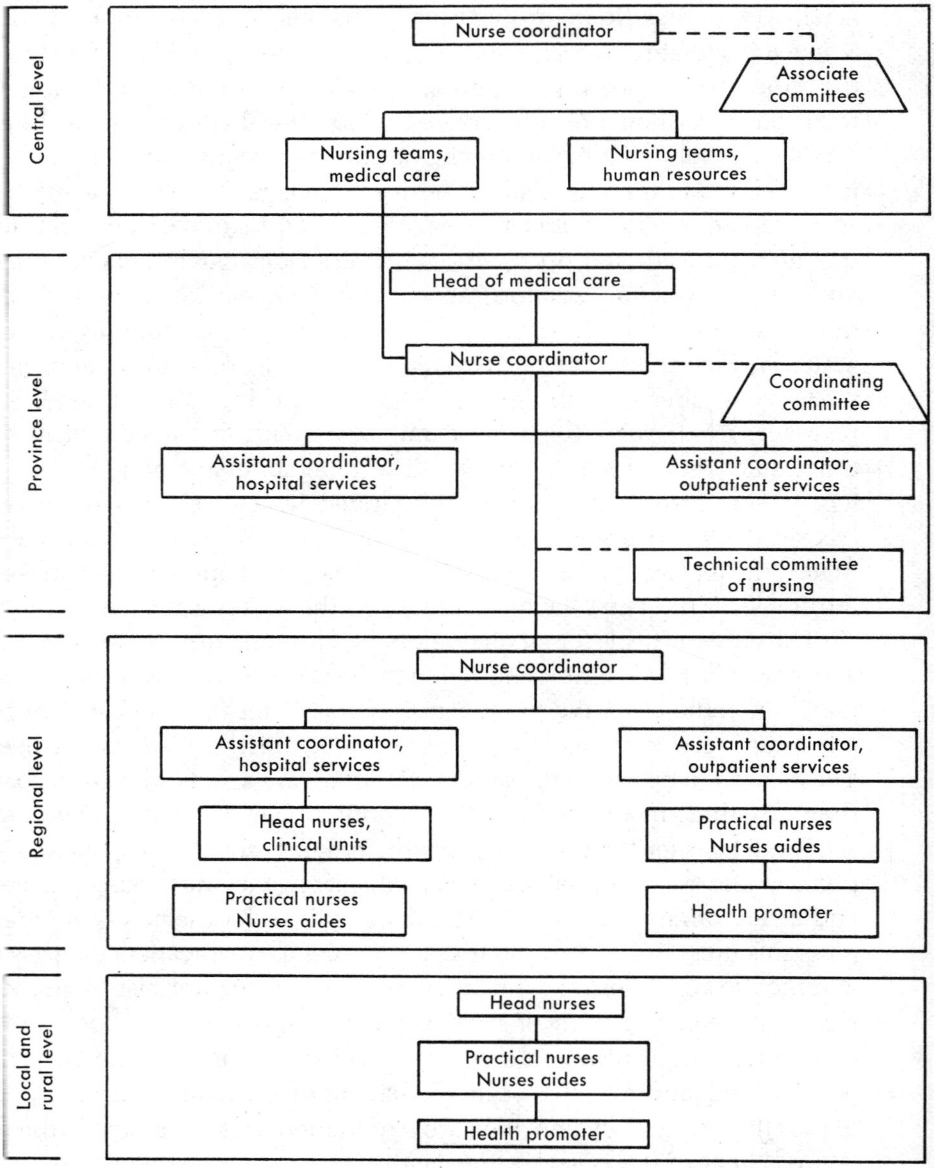

FIG. 11

Nursing services in Colombia. (Modified from Ministerio de Salud Publica: Estudio nacional de la situacion de enfermeria en Colombia, Republica de Colombia, 1972.)

bia. However, most universities have common criteria in the organization of their curricula, and courses include general, social, basic medical, and nursing sciences. The schools organize the content matter to meet the needs of the areas they serve.[15]

NURSING SERVICES

The organization of nursing services in Colombia is shown in Fig. 11.

Cuba

HEALTH SERVICES

Before the revolution of 1959, the social and economic conditions and the health patterns of the people of Cuba compared with those of other parts of Latin America. At present, although scarcity of health manpower exists, the health of the population of Cuba is better than that elsewhere in Latin America.[17] Primary health care in Cuba is made available to almost the entire population, in contrast to nonexistent health services in rural areas before 1959. Health policies and programs emphasize aspects of preventive, rehabilitative, and curative medicine; the planned collaboration between professional, auxiliary, and volunteer personnel; and active participation by the community in the arrangements of the health services.[2,17]

The Ministry of Health in Cuba is responsible for the Cuban health policy and for health administration, planning, and supervision. Primary, secondary, and tertiary care are available to the Cuban people at polyclinics, regional hospital centers, and provincial hospital centers, respectively. Nurses at the different care levels are grouped according to their specialties—adults, children, and public health. All health workers in Cuba belong to one union, regardless of their level of training or discipline.[17]

NURSING EDUCATION

Nursing education lasts for three and one-half years and requires completion of nine years of primary and secondary education. General education is integrated with nursing courses so that on graduation the nurses are at the preuniversity level. Most clinical experience of student nurses is in general or specialized hospitals, with a limited amount of experience in polyclinics and rural sections. After graduation the nurse is assigned to a special area of need for one or two years.

Postbasic education is available at the National Teaching Unit, which offers courses in epidemiology, nutrition, sanitation, and health services administration. For nurses, courses in obstetrical, pediatric, and adult nursing are offered along with administration and teaching. University-level nursing education is not yet available in Cuba, although some efforts are being made to establish a university-based degree program.[17]

Mexico

For centuries nursing in Mexico was done by sisterhoods and brotherhoods of the Catholic church. However, about the middle of the eighteenth century, the political revolution brought with it a decrease in the number of churches and, consequently, in the number of church officials, leading to a neglect in nursing practice. Nursing was taken over by the university of Mexico in 1911, and both nursing education and midwifery were placed under the supervision of the medical school.[27]

Modern nursing in Mexico, like that of other Latin American countries, came about as the result of cooperation among nurses, the government, and other national and international agencies such as the League of the Red Cross Societies, the Institute of Inter-American Affairs, and the Rockefeller Foundation. Of these groups, the Red Cross was responsible for introducing basic nursing education at the time of World War II. The Red Cross School of Nursing offers a three-year program in nursing and the University of Mexico School of Nursing has a four-year program. They are the best known schools among many of those that offer basic courses in nursing.[26]

In 1935 the University of Mexico School of Nursing, with the help of the Rockefeller Foundation, initiated the first graduate course in public health nursing. In addition, scholarships and fellowships were awarded by the Rockefeller Foundation to Mexican nurses for study in the United States. Some graduate nurses were also sent to the United States for one-year courses in administration, supervision, and teaching in hospitals and schools of nursing.[26]

MEXICAN NURSES' ASSOCIATION

The Mexican Nurses' Association became a reality in 1947. Its goal was to promote the educational and professional progress of Mexican nurses, translating this progress into better care for individuals, both well and sick, thus fulfilling the role that present-day society requires of nursing. The association was also interested in promoting and strengthening the bond between Mexican and foreign groups and maintaining a relationship with the International Council of Nurses. Following in-depth studies of the role of the nursing profession in the health care system, the *Colegio National de Enfermeras* was founded. It is a corporation of public right created by law, representing professional nurses before the public powers and authorities. The *Colegio* has intensified the goals set by the Mexican Nurses' Association.

The *Colegio National de Enfermeras* offers, not only to those who practice the profession but also to those who receive its benefits, all the advantages derived from such a status, which is reflected in the improvement of health care of the Mexican population.[16]

REFERENCES

1. Bareira, I.: Changes in the image of the nurse in Brazil, International Nursing Review **23:**43-47, March-April, 1976.
2. Beck, F.: Impressions of a visit to Latin America, International Nursing Review **6:**53-59, April, 1959.
3. Bullough, V., and Bullough, B.: The emergence of modern nursing, ed. 2, London, 1969, The Macmillan Co.
4. Chagas, A.: Modern nursing in Latin America, American Journal of Nursing **53:**34-36, 1953.
5. De Alcantara, G.: Nursing in Brazil, American Journal of Nursing **53:**576-579, 1953.
6. Development of nursing service in Brazil, American Journal of Nursing **22:** 560, 1922.
7. Dock, L., and Stewart, M.: A short history of nursing, New York, 1938, G. P. Putnam's Sons.
8. Goodnow, M.: Nursing history, ed. 9, Philadelphia, 1955, W. B. Saunders Co.
9. Guanes, H.: Nursing education in Brazil, International Nursing Review **5:** 32-33, 1958.
10. Hentsch, Y.: Nursing in Latin America, American Journal of Nursing **43:**440-442, 1943.
11. Jackson, J.: Nursing in Brazil, American Journal of Nursing **2:**56-57, 1901.
12. Jameison, E., Sewall, M., and Suhrie, E.: Trends in nursing history, ed. 6, Philadelphia, 1966, W. B. Saunders Co.
13. Jaramillo, A. A.: Historia y desarrollo de la enfermeria en Colombia, Revista de la Facultad de Medicina **17:**1075-1079, 1948.
14. Jensen, D. M.: History and trends of professional nursing, ed. 4, St. Louis, 1959, The C. V. Mosby Co.
15. Ministry of Health, Colombia: Nursing in the world, 1976, unpublished manuscript. (Available from the Ministerio De Salud Publica, Republica De Colombia.)
16. Moreno, G. T.: Mexican Nurses' Association: change for development, International Nursing Review **19:**(4):370-376, 1972.
17. Mussallem, H. K.: A glimpse of nursing in Cuba, Canadian Nurse **69:**23-30, 1973.
18. O'Hara, H.: Public health nursing in Latin America, Public Health Nursing **42:**73-78, 1950.
19. Parsons, E.: Modern nursing in Brazil, American Journal of Nursing **27:**443-449, 1927.
20. Ponte, M. L.: A rapid glance at Brazilian postgraduate education, International Journal of Nursing Studies **4:**37-46, 1967.
21. Progress in nursing education in Latin America, International Nursing Review **14:**64, Jan.-Feb., 1967.
22. Pullen, B.: Nursing in Brazil, American Journal of Nursing **35:**345-350, 1935.
23. Restrepo, R.: Nursing in Colombia, Canadian Nurse **65:**37, 1969.
24. Sellew, G., and Ebel, E.: A history of nursing, ed. 3, St. Louis, 1955, The C. V. Mosby Co.
25. Seymer, L. R.: A general history of nursing, London, 1932, Faber & Faber Ltd.
26. Stewart, I., and Austin, A.: A history of nursing, New York, 1962, G. P. Putnam's Sons.

27. Vasquez, S.: Nursing resources in Mexico, International Nursing Review **20:** 20-24, Jan.-Feb., 1973.
28. Wood, B.: Nursing in Brazil, Nursing Times **24:**266-267, 1928.

PART IV

Near and Middle East

Chapter 15

LEBANON

In the early days when sickness or a confinement occurred in a Lebanese family, one of the more experienced women of the community, or the mother, sister, cousin, or aunt, cared for the sick person. The old midwife had considerable influence on the care of the sick, especially if the patient was a woman or child. Lack of nursing personnel constituted a great difficulty in the care of the sick. Although the work of Florence Nightingale in the Crimean War and her contributions to the development of modern nursing were known to the Lebanese people, a long time elapsed before nursing was established and recognized as a profession.[6]

A simple form of nursing was begun in Beirut in 1847 by the French Sisters of Charity of the Order of St. Vincent de Paul.[1] They ministered to the sick in a small hospital attached to their convent. In 1860 the Prussian Knights of the Order of St. John built a hospital in Beirut, which was later called the French Military Hospital. In this hospital, nursing was done by German deaconesses of the Kaiserwerth Sisterhood, who later trained some Lebanese and Syrian nurses to serve as assistant nurses in their hospital. These episodes marked the beginning of nursing in that part of the world.[6]

BEGINNING OF MODERN NURSING

Modern training of nurses in the country was the outcome of the establishment of the school of nursing in 1905 in connection with the American University of Beirut.[10] The school has been the center of training for Syrian and Lebanese probationers, whose certificate was recognized for higher posts. Previously, a few isolated nurses provided care. They were either foreigners or Syrians, some of whom received their training abroad, whereas the rest were trained by missionary hospitals in Lebanon.[6,7]

Adla Wartabet was one of the first nurses to come to Beirut after receiving her degree under the Nightingale system in England. In 1900 she took charge of the Greek Orthodox Hospital of St. George, where she served for three years. Many other Lebanese nurses went abroad to study nursing as early as 1875, with the intention of starting a school to train nurses in Lebanon on their return and hence render service to their own people. Evidently, a great need for a school of nursing existed, and this was met by the inauguration of the American University of Beirut School of Nursing. The school was designed to meet the needs of Asia Minor, Syria, and Egypt for the education of nurses. Jane E. Van Zandt, a graduate of the New York Postgraduate Hospital, was put in charge of the school. A Mrs. Dale was appointed superintendent of the hospital and was responsible for the clinical part of the instruction.[6,7]

The enrollment of Lebanese women at the school was not high for several years because parents preferred that their daughters remain at home or marry and considered that a young woman's dignity was lowered by serving in a hospital. Also, the education of young Lebanese women early in the century was not generally recognized. However, if a girl needed to earn her living, teaching was almost always preferred. Many young refugee Armenian women who had been educated in orphanages or by relief funds needed to work for a living in Lebanon.[9]

The first three-year program required an elementary education and some knowledge of English for admission. Instruction was in English by professors of the College of Medicine. In 1928 the school adopted the same standards for nursing education that were developed in New York State, and in 1932 a high school diploma was required for admission into the school of nursing. This change resulted in approval of the school by the New York State Board of Nurse Examiners of the State Education Department, which later led to its approval by the Lebanese Ministry of Education.[8]

NURSING EDUCATION

The American University of Beirut School of Nursing offers two programs, a diploma in nursing, which is being phased out in line with recent developments in nursing, and a bachelor of science degree. The bachelor of science program began in 1936 as a two-year liberal arts curriculum followed by three years of nursing. This program was changed in 1964 to offer an integrated course of study in nursing, science, and liberal arts over four calendar years. Lebanese students should have the government certificate, Baccalaureate Part II in Science, to be accepted. This reduces the program to three years, since the government certificate is equivalent to a university freshman level.

In 1952 two postbasic programs for diploma graduates were established at the American University of Beirut School of Nursing to serve the needs of graduate nurses from Middle Eastern and African countries. One program focuses on public health nursing, and the other prepares teachers and nursing service administrators with clinical specialties in medical-surgical, maternal and child health, or psychiatric nursing. A third program was recently started for nurse-midwives seeking preparation as tutors in midwifery.[8]

Between 1933 and 1973 other nursing schools were established, mostly private. Eleven schools presently prepare professional nurses. Nine are private, one is government, and one is a program in psychiatric nursing. Only two of these programs lead to a bachelor of science degree and a license. They are offered at the American University of Beirut and the French University, respectively. Throughout the country nursing classes are held in Arabic, English, and French. A constant exchange of ideas between the schools is made possible through regular meetings of the directors of the schools or through frequent seminars and workshops to study problems facing nursing educators.[8]

Classroom and clinical instruction in all the schools is done by nurses, providing a continuity for the learner. However, physicians are invited frequently to lecture on topics in medicine. The fact that nursing textbooks are mainly available in French and English limits enrollment of student nurses who are not fluent in either language.

NURSING PROGRAMS

The country now has three programs of nursing. The first is the four-year, university-based professional nurse program, which requires students to have passed the Baccalaureate Part II certificate, the government examination. The second program is based on the Ministry of Education Law, passed in 1966, which requires a minimum of eleven years of general education followed by three or more years of nursing education in a recognized school of nursing and which leads to a diploma in nursing. The third program is more recent and resulted from the 1968 Ministry of Education Law, which established a technical nurse program similar to the pattern of European technical programs. The student in this program enters with ten years of education and the Brevet Certificate, a government certificate, and after two years receives the technical Baccalaureate Part I in Nursing. At the end of two years of general education, science, and nursing, followed by a government examination, the Technical Baccalaureate Part II in Nursing is granted.[5,8]

The French Faculty of Medicine School of Nursing was established in 1938 as a school for midwifery and nursing. In 1942 it was separated into two schools, one for midwives and the other for general nurses. The Baccalaureate Part II certificate is required for entry to the school, which offers a three-year program at the end of which the student receives the "license" in nursing. In 1945 the Red Cross School of Nursing was founded in Beirut. It requires its students to carry the Baccalaureate Part I certificate. After three years in nursing and general education studies, the student has to sit for the Technical Baccalaureate Part II examination.[8]

Practical nursing programs, varying from six to twelve months, are offered at the American University Hospital, the Red Cross, the National School of Nursing, and Hôtel Dieu. The student is required to have the Brevet certificate for entrance. These programs have contributed to better nursing care than that previously done in most hospitals by aides.

Graduate-level nursing education is still lacking in Lebanon. Present efforts concentrate on establishing a master's of science program at the American University of Beirut. Nurses who wish to pursue graduate-level education currently go to the United States or Europe. Continuing education is a growing field in Lebanon, and Lebanese nurses from different schools cooperate in planning seminars, workshops, and short refresher courses for nurses in the region.[8]

In addition to the general nursing courses in different nursing schools in Lebanon, a three-year course in psychiatric nursing is offered at the Lebanese Hospital for Mental and Nervous Disorders. This hospital, which is unique in the Middle East, was established in 1900 by Theophilus Waldmeier, a pastor and missionary. Training of students was in English, and later a course in Arabic was started. This school admits students who are sent by their governments from different countries in the area. Standards of training followed the British system at the beginning but were changed gradually to meet the country's nursing needs.[4]

The Maternity and Child Health Center was opened in Beirut in 1951 as a result of an agreement between the government of Lebanon, the World Health Organization, and UNICEF.[2] With the plan to advance maternity and child health care in the area, Mary Mango, a World Health Organization public health nurse and midwife, was assigned to the center to help the Lebanese staff in the training of maternal and child health nurses. The maternity services performed by the nurses proved to be effective in promoting the health of mothers and children.[3]

NURSING ORGANIZATION

In view of the tremendous complexity concerning nonprofessional groups in the nursing profession who were licensed at an earlier time, Lebanese nurses are still struggling to establish an association that will group the graduate nurses together. The establishment of such an order would require all registered nurses to join in order to practice and will help in the development of nursing as a profession in the country. Nurses representing the various schools that form the Central Committee of Nursing are currently working with the Ministries of Health and Education to speed up the process. Membership in the International Council of Nurses was granted to Lebanese nurses in 1969.[8]

NURSING CONDITIONS

About 95.5% of the registered nurses in Lebanon in 1970 were women.[5] At present more male nurses are being trained, but many of them migrate to work as nurses in neighboring Arab countries where the pay is greater. Many female registered nurses in Lebanon are not actually practicing nursing; some marry and leave their jobs, whereas others emigrate to other countries where working conditions are more appealing. This leaves the country in constant need of more trained nurses. To attract the inactive group of nurses back to the profession, the government has been working on better salary scales, fringe benefits, and working hours as a step in meeting the needs of the people.

REFERENCES

1. Cardwell, V.: Public health nursing in Lebanon, Public Health Nursing **35:**430-434, 1943.
2. Edwards, M.: Health services in Lebanon, Nursing Times **60:**848, 1964.
3. Mango, M.: British nurse-midwife with WHO, Nursing Mirror **99:**iv-v, June 26, 1954.
4. Mitchell, A.: Unique mental hospital in the Middle East, Nursing Mirror **99:** viii-ix, April 23, 1954.
5. Rifka, G. E.: Nursing manpower in Lebanon, International Nursing Review **17**(3):195-205, 1970.
6. Shahla, S.: Nursing in Syria, American Journal of Nursing **30:**1515-1518, 1930.
7. Stevens, E.: Nursing in Syria, Nursing Times **23:**1063, 1927.
8. Thomas, G. M.: Nursing in Lebanon, International Nursing Review **22:**138-143, Sept.-Oct., 1975.
9. Van Zandt, J.: A training school of nurses in the Turkish Empire, American Journal of Nursing **9:**274-276, 1909.
10. Watt, C.: Visiting eleven countries, Nursing Times **46:**761-762, 1950.

Chapter 16

ISRAEL

Israel, formerly called Palestine, had several mission hospitals under German deaconesses, French religious sisters, Scottish, and English nurses. Some young Palestinian women studied nursing, but the majority were secluded and seldom showed interest in a profession that was not highly regarded by the public.[8,10] In 1912 a small group of Jewish women in New York, organized under the name Hadassah, took an interest in the health conditions in Palestine and as a result sent two American nurses to Jerusalem early in 1913. These nurses devoted themselves mainly to maternity care, which included organization and supervision of midwives, and to district visiting nursing.[13]

Most of the welfare activities in Palestine before World War I were maintained by foreign agencies. During the war many of these agencies ceased to function, and as a result, a number of hospitals were closed. Toward the end of the war, health conditions became desperate because of famine, the primitive sanitary conditions, and a shortage of physicians and nurses.[11] Epidemics of infectious diseases spread over the country, killing and disabling many people. Following an appeal by local authorities, Hadassah sent to Palestine a unit of physicians, nurses, and sanitary engineers with a large supply of drugs. This unit in 1918 opened hospitals and clinics in Jerusalem, Jaffa, Tiberias, and Safad and expanded rapidly into a countrywide system that included dispensaries, health welfare centers, and other allied educational and preventive activities.[6,13] Under direction of a Dr. Finley, the American Red Cross society sent a medical and social service unit to Palestine to meet the devastating hospital needs of the country.[12]

BEGINNING OF NURSING EDUCATION

The Hadassah School of Nursing was established within three months of the arrival of the medical team in Palestine. The school was attached to the Rothschild Hospital in Jerusalem and offered a three-year nursing course. The studies included anatomy, materia media, theory of nursing, dietetics, bacteriology, hygiene, and medical-surgical, obstetrical, and pediatric nursing. Clinical training in each nursing area was provided in the various hospitals of the country and extended over a period of three months. The Gymnasium, a high school diploma, was required for admission, as well as fluency in the Hebrew language.[2,6]

Each year a postgraduate course was offered in public health nursing to graduate nurses who showed an interest in pursuing further study and an aptitude in the work. The course included district maternity nursing, prenatal and postnatal care, infant welfare and preschool nursing, and tuberculosis nursing. Many nurses also were sent to the United States to specialize in teaching and administration so that they could take over when the American nurses had to leave.[6,13]

Between 1934 and 1946, seven schools of nursing were operating under Hebrew auspices. In the meantime the Department of Health of the British Mandatory Government had opened hospitals for the Arab-Palestinian population. British-trained nurses headed these hospitals and conducted short nursing courses to teach nursing and midwifery to local young women. As a result, the standard colonial nursing curriculum was introduced to these hospitals in Palestine.[7,14]

When Israel was formed in 1948, Israeli nurses stepped into administrative and teaching positions, and the new Ministry of Health established a division of nursing headed by a Hadassah graduate nurse. Nursing leaders were then trying to establish standards for nursing care and nursing education, especially after the great influx of refugees who claimed to be nurses but who had no documents to prove it. The International Council of Nurses, through a London office, opened to help war-torn nurses establish their identity. They helped the nurses of Israel by cooperating closely with the nursing division in the Ministry of Health to verify the nursing education claimed by the new immigrant nurses. Israel became a member of the International Council of Nurses in 1965.[16]

NURSING EDUCATION TODAY

Today seventeen schools of professional nursing in Israel offer a three-year hospital program comparable with the diploma program in the United States. Public health nursing is greatly emphasized in the curriculum of these schools, since it is viewed as one of the most important functions of nurses.[5] Work and study at community health centers comprise an integral part of the curriculum. Students are given the opportunity to observe families in their homes and study the dynamics that affect the family's structure. At completion of the three-year program, students are awarded the diploma of State Registered Nurse. Postbasic educational programs in public health nursing, midwifery, operating-room techniques, and mental health nursing are available to nurses who wish to pursue higher education. The programs are six to twelve months long, depending on the area of study, and graduates become specialists in their own fields.[9,16]

A program leading to the baccalaureate degree in nursing was recently started at the Hebrew University, including two years of academic study in chemistry, biochemistry, physics, sociology, anatomy and physiology, social welfare, and occupational therapy. During this time introductory courses to nursing practice are given, accompanied by ward visits once a week. This is followed by two years of nursing courses and internship in a specialty area. To deal with the problems of staff advancement that might accompany such a program, the director of the school of nursing equated ten years of head-nurse experience with a bachelor's degree.[9]

Practical nursing programs are also available in Israel and usually admit students who have finished eight years of schooling. The program lasts for eighteen months, during which students are trained to do simple nursing procedures and to assist graduate nurses in carrying out the unit work. Programs to prepare nurses' aids are also available throughout the country.[16]

KIBBUTZ NURSING

A typical feature of nursing in Israel is the kibbutz nurse who works in a kibbutz and is a member. The nurse may have joined the kibbutz voluntarily, married into it, or have been born to it and hence sent by it to a nursing school. The nurse's main functions include general and public health nursing, which are offered in the framework of the community. Like other members, the nurse lives on a collective farm, sharing the work, income, and general activities of the kibbutz. Nursing covers the full range, from clinic work to bedside care and health teaching.[15]

NURSING ORGANIZATION

Most professional groups in Israel, including the National Association of Nurses in Israel (NANI), are members of *Histadrut,* the National Labor Organization. NANI is the negotiating body for wages, hours of work, and working conditions. Activities such as curriculum planning and nursing legislation are the responsibilities of the Ministry of Health with which NANI participates and has a great deal of influential power. Nursing communication with other professional associations is facilitated by joint membership in the *Histadrut.* Various professional groups meet regularly in service team conferences and cooperate on health matters. The medical group tends to be paternalistic in Israel, as in most other countries. However, nurses are struggling to overcome this subservience and antagonism to the medical staff and to cooperate on an equal level. In the health service organizations, nursing is in a good position to communicate effectively because of the availability of nursing leadership at every level, including the Ministry of Health.[1,3]

PRIMARY HEALTH CARE

In the overall delivery of health care services, outpatient care is stressed. Minor surgery and complicated treatments are performed on an outpatient basis because of the proximity and access to these facilities. Moreoever, community health centers located in every part of the nation stress prevention, provide maternal and child health care, and offer different services depending on the needs of the community. Public health nurses do home visits to educate the family about the importance of prevention and about the availability of outpatient facilities that provide primary care needs.[4]

REFERENCES

1. Bergman, R.: Nursing and organized groups in society, International Nursing Review **12:**28-31, Dec., 1965.
2. Bergman, R.: Israel's educators in the diploma schools of nursing, International Journal of Nursing Studies **8:**103-126, 1971.
3. Bergman, R.: Opinion on nursing, International Nursing Review **18**(2):195-230, 1971.
4. Bergman, R.: Opinion on nursing, International Nursing Review **23**(1):15-24, 1976.
5. Bergman, R.: Team nursing in public health Israel, International Journal of Nursing Studies **2:**261-267, 1965.
6. Bluestone, M.: The Hadassah School of Nursing, American Journal of Nursing **28:**1093-1097, 1928.
7. Cantor, S.: Nursing in Israel, American Journal of Nursing **51:**162-163, 1951.
8. Dock, L., and Stewart, I.: A short history of nursing, New York, 1938. G. P. Putnam's Sons.
9. Golub, S.: Nursing in Israel, Nursing Mirror **136:**22-25, June 15, 1973.
10. Goodnow, M.: Nursing history, ed. 9, Philadelphia, 1955, W. B. Saunders Co.
11. Harefooah: Palestine's first medical journal, American Journal of Nursing **20:** 980, 1920.
12. Noyes, C.: The Red Cross, American Journal of Nursing **19:**367-376, 1919.
13. Selisberg, A.: A modern training school for nurses in Jerusalem, American Journal of Nursing **21:**721-723, 1921.
14. Shulamith, L.: A nursing school in Palestine, American Journal of Nursing **40:**880-884, 1940.
15. Weiss, O.: Kibbutz nurses, American Journal of Nursing **71:**1762-1765, 1971.
16. Weiss, Q.: Nurses and nursing in Israel, Nursing Outlook **14:**58-60, 1966.

Chapter 17

IRAN

In past centuries Persia, now known as Iran, had government hospitals in its chief cities that were staffed with paid attendants. Later, the fatalistic attitude of the Moslem religion slackened the interest of the government, which resulted in neglect of the sick. In the middle of the nineteenth century, however, American missionaries demonstrated great interest in the area and, as a result, began medical work by gradually establishing hospitals in several cities. Also, American and British church missionaries opened some schools of nursing, the oldest of which were at Tehran and Tabriz, started as early as 1916. In spite of the availability of schools of nursing, a lack of qualified applicants existed for a long time. Women were secluded, and girls did not have sufficient education at the high school level.[2]

DEVELOPMENT OF MODERN NURSING

The abolition of the veil was ordered in January, 1936, and women were encouraged to find themselves a career or profession outside the home. This remarkable change opened an avenue for the development of modern nursing in Iran. As a result, three schools of nursing were opened in Tehran, Tabriz, and Meshed. Since the Minister of Education was familiar with nursing education in the United States, American nurses were recruited to organize these schools. In 1937 the Board of Foreign Missions of the Presbyterian Church asked three nurse educators to go to Iran to help organize the new schools of nursing. The course of study in these government schools was two years; students admitted had received nine years of general education. To raise the prestige of nurses in the country, graduates of these schools were called physician's assistants.[5,9]

After World War II the Imperial Foundation under the sponsorship of the royal family began the task of improving nursing conditions in Iran. As a result, the Princess Ashraf School of Nursing was built, and British nurses were appointed to teach in it. The admission requirement was eleven or twelve years of general education. To be more prestigious, the school of nursing affiliated with the University of Tehran Medical School—an accomplishment that advanced nursing education.[5] The establishment of a nursing school by the Red-Lion-and-Sun Organization, known as the Iranian Red Cross, was further evidence of the awakening interest in the profession. The teaching staff of this school was greatly assisted by the World Health Organization nursing education department.[5]

PUBLIC HEALTH PROGRAMS

Iran's generalized public health program was started in 1951 under the direction of American nurses and the American Point Four Program. The foremost aim of such a program was the training of public health nurses in a two-year course that prepared them to instruct the villagers about personal and community health, nutrition, maternal and child health, and communicable diseases. The curriculum of such programs included clinical and bedside nursing care as well as theoretical work. The American nurses at first took complete charge of nursing activities. In time, however, as Iranian nurses gained more experience, more responsibilities were delegated to them.[1,8] In response to the severe shortage of nurses, midwives were recruited who, because of their good preparation, accomplished pioneer work in the public health field in Iran.[8]

NURSING DIVISION

In 1952 the Ministry of Health approved the establishment of a nursing unit, which later became the nursing division. This recognition has helped Iranian nurses receive deserved recognition as a profession. The division consisted of four sections, each with its own consultant in the fields of public health, nursing education, hospital nursing service administration, and nursing resources and registration. The division set standards defining the education of nurses and the services of nurse educators. Assistance was also given to school administrators in developing their policies, in planning and implementing curricula, and in improving methods of testing and evaluation.[5]

NURSING EDUCATION

Nurses from Iran attended the First Grand Nursing Conference in 1956. It was planned following the recommendation of the Ninth World Health Assembly, which emphasized that individual countries should review and evaluate their nursing programs to improve the status of nursing and the care of the sick. As a result of this conference, constitutions for professional and practical nursing schools were drafted and approved by the Council of Education in 1958. This movement led to the raising of professional requirements for schools of nursing to the twelfth grade of general education and to the extension of the program to cover three calendar years. The requirement for practical nursing schools was set at the ninth grade of general education to enter a two-year course of study.[5] The Nemazee School of Nursing, founded in 1954, was the first school in Iran to require the minimum twelve years of general education for its applicants. It was also the first school to give the certificate of "License" in English to its graduates.[4]

The first school to offer the four-year course in nursing, leading to the bachelor of nursing science degree, was established in 1965 by the World Health Organization. Other schools were later established that included in their curriculum general college courses as well as nursing courses. As part of an overall plan for the development of advanced nursing education, this program provided an opportunity for registered nurses who were interested in teaching and supervision positions to seek a bachelor's degree in nursing. Instruction is in English, and the program usually requires five semesters. The creation of this university-level postbasic program has opened the possibility for nursing to develop in harmony with related sciences.[3-5]

Preparation beyond the basic nursing programs in Iran became available for the first time in 1954 as midwifery training. Prior to that time a midwife was not required to be a nurse. The basic midwifery course earlier was offered by the University of Tehran over a three-year period. However, this training course was changed to a twelve-month postbasic program in 1954 and is still offered at the University of Tehran to graduate nurses. Scholarships were also made available to graduate nurses who were interested in seeking graduate education in foreign countries. Many nurses went to Lebanon seeking either the bachelor's degree in nursing or the master's degree in public health, both of which are offered at the American University of Beirut. Other nurses were sent to England or the United States for further nursing study or specialization.[5,7]

IRANIAN HEALTH CORPS

The shortage of trained health personnel exists in most countries of the world and especially in the underdeveloped and developing countries. To provide health care facilities to the rural areas, which have 60% of the population, the Iranian government established the Iranian Health Corps, into which most medical graduates and some high school graduates are inducted instead of the regular military service. However, this program has been unable to expand into a comprehensive health care system because many of these physicians and their assistants, after the two-year draft period, choose to practice in urban rather than rural areas. To remedy this problem, the primary level health worker was introduced into the health system. Trainee candidates admitted into the programs should have six years of general schooling, should be no less than 18 years of age, and should live in the areas where they are to serve. The curricula of these programs are designed in accordance with the needs of the rural areas and are six months long.[6]

This project, derived from observing the functions of the Chinese barefoot doctor, is designed to follow such models in different countries in which village authorities participate in the selection of candidates to be trained as auxiliary health workers. These workers would live and work in their own villages. On graduation from the program the health workers spend from 1 to 6 hours a day in a clinic, during which time they see and treat patients, sometimes referring them to the health corps station physician. Patients are also instructed about preventive measures to obviate a return visit. Through the follow-up home and village visits, the workers discuss with villagers, either individually or in groups, family planning, sanitation, and nutrition. A full-time physician is responsible for the work done at the clinic and usually checks on the health workers at least once a week.[6]

Iran, like other developing countries, is faced with difficulties in its attempts to establish an effective health care delivery system. Easing the manpower shortage seems to be the most critical step at present in providing better health care for the people.

REFERENCES

1. Aftab, S.: Nursing and Point Four in Iran, Nursing World **127:**8-10, 1953.
2. Goodnow, M.: Nursing history, ed. 9, Philadelphia, 1955, W. B. Saunders Co.
3. Kelly, M. A.: Beliefs of Iranian nurses and nursing students about nurses and nursing education, International Nursing Review **20:**108-111, July-Aug., 1973.
4. Moghadassy, M.: Progress: postbasic nursing education in Iran, International Nursing Review **19**(1):3-11, 1972.
5. Riahi, A.: Nursing education in Iran, International Journal of Nursing Studies **5:**267-271, 1968.
6. Ronaghy, H. A.: The front line health worker: selection, training, and performance, American Journal of Public Health **66**(3):273-277, 1976.
7. Ronaghy, H. A.: Migration of Iranian nurses to the United States: a study of one school of nursing in Iran, International Nursing Review **22**(3):87-88, 1975.
8. Salsali, A.: Iran's nurses, American Journal of Nursing **61:**99, 1961.
9. Setzler, L.: In Iran, American Journal of Nursing **41:**520-525, 1941.

Chapter 18

INDIA

India's religions, Hinduism and Moslemism, hampered the progress of nursing in that country for a long time, since they discouraged interference with existing conditions. Also, the low status of women, the seclusion of Moslem women, racial prejudice, general illiteracy, and poverty played a part in hindering attempts to develop a good health care system.[9] Before the Western powers in general and the English in particular established rule in India, Christian missionaries did the first skilled nursing in India, establishing hospitals to provide medical relief. During the latter part of the nineteenth century, missionary nurses who came to India from England, Australia, France, and the United States worked hard to establish missionary centers, which in many cases served as health clinics for treating and teaching the public.[1,10]

The Lady Dufferin Fund, established in 1885 and now administered by the government, began by educating women physicians, which was extended later to nurses. Earlier, foreign women physicians and nurses cared for female patients, who were not allowed to be examined by male physicians. The establishment of the British rule gave impetus to the establishment of medical services, which were patterned after those of European countries.[16] Other Western powers, such as France and Portugal, also influenced nursing and medical practices in India. Their influences merged with the traditional beliefs and practices of the natives of India, leading to health services that were patterned after those of the various countries.[1,6]

The first two nursing schools were established at Madras and Bombay in 1884 and 1886, respectively. During the same period a number of missionary hospitals organized short nursing courses. Soon, schools of nursing patterned along the lines of the Western countries were established throughout the country, and nursing education advanced beyond that offered in Calcutta, Madras, and Bombay, which formed the bases of administration of the British rule. From that time on a gradual extension of modern nursing in India took place, in spite of the fact that difficulties of religious and racial customs and political conditions had been greater there than in any other part of the world.[1,10]

NURSING DEVELOPMENTS

The year 1943 marked an awakening that had great influence on the practice of nursing in India. With World War II at its height and freedom within sight, the realization came that the departure of the British nurses would have a tremendous impact on nursing administration. British nurses, at the time, constituted most of the nursing teachers and matrons of the country. The Indian Military Nursing Service, seeing the realities of the situation, persuaded the government to make provisions for the preparation of Indian nurses for administration and teaching posts. This movement provided sufficient impetus among government officials to start the first post-certificate School of Administration in Delhi. Gradually the idea caught on. The Civil Nursing Services took advantage of the situation and instituted a course for nurses who were interested in teaching. Scholarships for both courses were made available through government agencies, the Indian Red Cross, and the Minto Nursing Association.[8,12]

THE BHORE REPORT

The appointment of the Health Survey and Development Committee was another highlight of 1943. This committee was given the task of surveying the health services of India and recommending the development of programs in the field.[8] The report of the committee, known as the *Bhore Report,* was published in 1946. It was a blueprint of the health needs of the people, recommending ways and means of meeting the overwhelming magnitude of existing health problems. The report described nursing conditions as deplorable and stressed the importance of having educated Indian women join the profession to raise its standards.[8]

The establishment of the two baccalaureate programs in nursing at the College of Nursing in Delhi and at the School of Nursing in Lahore were direct outcomes of the *Bhore Report.* The course proved to be valuable in encouraging a group of educated women to join the profession in spite of family resistance that viewed nursing as the job of the low caste.[7,20] These programs integrated academic work and nursing courses throughout a carefully planned four-year program.

Male nurses played an important role in the health care programs of India. This fact is attributed to the social conditions and customs of the country, which give men more freedom than women. As a result, men could go out to nurse in districts where women were not permitted. Another outcome of the *Bhore Report* was the recruitment and training of male nurses so that they could be employed to a greater extent in male wards and male outpatient clinics of government hospitals.[1]

THE INDIAN NURSING COUNCIL

The Indian Nursing Council Act of 1947 was the predecessor for the National Nursing Council, established in 1959 as a result of the recommendation of the Bhore Committee. The main purpose behind the National Nursing Council was to bring about uniformity in nursing education.[1,3] The first five-year plan, started in 1950, emphasized the development of public health services and hence the training of personnel to serve in the different areas. The World Health Organization and UNICEF provided advisors, equipment, and personnel to help start a nationwide public health campaign. Soon Indian and international teams were working side by side to combat the spread of infectious diseases that were prevalent in the postwar period.[7] In the meantime many one-year courses were made available in pediatrics, tuberculosis, public health, and psychiatric nursing for graduate nurses immediately involved in these areas.[7,21]

PRIMARY HEALTH CARE

In 1952 the integration of medical and public health services at all levels and the establishment of primary health centers were launched by the government. These centers catered for both preventive and curative services by providing personal and informal care to the rural population. Health education, antenatal and postnatal care, family planning, child health care, and home visits comprised most of the activities of primary health centers.[13] In addition, the Red Cross society of India, having the cooperation of the upper classes, sponsored two-year training courses for health visitors, including midwifery. Graduates of these courses worked in rural areas, teaching and promoting health care among Indian people.[18,21]

NURSING EDUCATION

As in the case of basic education, India also had an early start in post-certificate education. Courses that are presently available include ward administration, pediatric nursing, midwifery, nursing education, and nursing school administration. All students are required to take the three-month ward administration course, which is followed by seven months in any one of the other areas. However, a revision of the program leading to the nurse tutor degree is indicated. It will include more emphasis on science and nursing. There also is a trend to integrate these courses into the baccalaureate program and provide specialization at the master's level.[4,14] A post-certificate course in public health nursing was added as a result of government emphasis on the expansion of health services in the country. Many courses were developed in this area that gained international importance, attracting candidates from the southeast Asia region.

As mentioned earlier, university education in nursing in India started as early as 1946. The colleges offer a four-year program leading to the Bachelor of Science degree (Honours) in nursing and qualifying students in general nursing, public health nursing, and midwifery.[15] Although the curriculum is modeled after the United States system, some adaptation to the conditions in India focus on the curative and preventive aspects of nursing and to a greater extent on family planning, which constitutes a major national objective in the health care delivery system of India. All graduates of the baccalaureate programs are exempted from the government's final examination, since the university's examinations are honored for registration and licensure.[5,14] In addition to the Bachelor of Science degree in nursing, diploma programs are still widely available in India.

Postgraduate education in nursing is relatively new in India. For many years nurses were sent abroad for study on the advanced level. The first master's program in nursing was established in 1959 at the University of Delhi. Another program was established ten years later in South India at the College of Nursing in Vellore, which is affiliated with the University of Madras. The general aim of these and other programs is the development of advanced competence in professional nursing, with emphasis on specialization in a major clinical area as well as on teaching and administration. Field experience in the three areas is provided, with special attention given to teaching in the clinical areas. An innovation in the graduate program is the introduction of a course on international health and nursing whose main purpose is to develop further understanding of international health and nursing activities, particularly the administration and organization of programs at the international level.[4,14]

A course for auxiliary nurse-midwives is available also to prepare candidates to staff the rural health centers. This two-year course includes nine months of general nursing and fifteen months of midwifery. On completion of the course, graduates work as midwives in primary health centers. Auxiliary nurse-midwives can take general nursing with six months' exemption from the total length of study, a provision made possible by the Indian Nursing Council.[1] Following the tradition of England, the health visitors' course was established by the Indian government. A two- and one-half year program, it prepares candidates for the health visitor certificate. Graduates are employed in maternity and child health clinics to supervise the work of auxiliary nurse-midwives. Health visitors can have an overall one-year exemption if they decide to take general nursing, on the condition that they meet the entrance requirements. Both auxiliary nurse-midwives and health visitors are increasingly utilized in India in family planning work—a role considered to be of prime importance for the Indian national health program.[2,17,19]

NURSING ASSOCIATIONS

The official nursing associations in India are similar to those of the English-speaking countries. The two recognized nursing organizations are the Trained Nurses' Association of India and the Association of Nursing

Superintendents.[10] Nursing registration began in 1923 as a result of efforts by the Trained Nurses' Association. The same association edits the *Indian Journal of Nursing,* which compares favorably with some of the nursing journals in the world. With the work of the organizations and the enthusiasm of the nurses, India has made important achievements in its nursing world.

PUBLIC HEALTH NURSING

The impetus to the development of public health nursing started with the development of the community health programs and primary health centers. In addition, the Bhore committee saw that the work done by the health visitors was insufficient to meet the needs of the country and to reach all sections of the population. At least four categories of staff presently comprise the public health team in India as follows:

1. The public health nurse who has had a postcertificate course in public health nursing or a bachelor of science degree in nursing recognized by the Indian Nursing Council
2. The nurse who has had a short course in public health nursing or has had public health integrated in the basic course
3. The health visitor
4. The auxiliary nurse-midwife

Supervision of the nursing staff in the public health field is done by health nursing supervisors who are assigned to every district in the country.[11]

INTERNATIONAL AID

International agencies have contributed considerably to the advancement of nursing in India during the last ten years. Aid in the form of fellowships and stipends, teaching and hospital equipment, and nursing teachers were provided by the different agencies. Fellowships for study abroad have given nurses the opportunity to specialize in a particular field of study or to qualify as teachers or administrators. Stipends made available by UNICEF have enabled a number of midwives and public health nurses to join the profession and have given the courses a good start by assuring a steady flow of students. The aid received from UNICEF was used in planning refresher courses that made it possible to bring nurses together from all parts of the country and to update them on their particular field of nursing. This has also provided a means to plan curricula in line with revised syllabi and to develop a more uniform pattern of nursing education.[11]

In addition, UNICEF has supplied schools of nursing with teaching equipment and supplies, which have contributed to the improvement in teaching programs. Also, equipment provided to hospitals, health centers, and clinics has helped in raising the morale of health workers by giving them good tools with which to work.[11]

The most valuable of all the work given to India by international agencies has been the contribution of the international nurses. Nurses from the World Health Organization have helped in various projects such as malaria, tuberculosis, venereal diseases, maternal and child health, mental health, nursing administration, and nursing education. In addition, nurses assigned through the United States Agency for International Development have helped to develop nursing at the state and central levels by establishing collegiate courses in nursing. Nurses under the Colombo Plan have also had their share in developing college-level teaching programs.[11]

NURSING SERVICE

Indian nurses are presently working in all branches of the health care delivery system, such as hospitals, health centers, sanatoria, industry, control programs for communicable diseases, and in private schools and schools for nurses. Some 95% of all nurses and midwives are employed by hospitals and nursing schools, whereas almost all health visitors and auxiliary nurse-midwives are employed by maternal and child health clinics and primary health centers. This trend is changing, since all nurses will be required to work in primary health centers when they are asked to do so.[11]

REFERENCES

1. Ahad, M. A.: Nursing education in India, International Nursing Review **17**(3): 224-237, 1970.
2. Bachu, A.: The nurse's role in family planning services in India, International Nursing Review **23**(1):25-28, 1976.
3. Bachu, A.: Indian nurses in I.S.A., International Nursing Review **20:**114-116, July-Aug., 1973.
4. Bachu, A.: Problems of nursing education in India in an age of technology, International Nursing Review **18**(1):85-95, 1971.
5. Bauman, M. B.: Baccalaureate nursing in a selected number of English speaking countries, International Nursing Review **9**(1):12-38, 1972.
6. Burnett, D.: A nurse visitor in India, Public Health Nursing **43:**408-412, 1951.
7. Devi, L.: Programs for India's graduate nurses, American Journal of Nursing **56:**334, 1956.
8. Devi, L.: Twelve years of nursing in India, International Nursing Review **2:**49-52, Oct., 1955.
9. Dock, L.: India, American Journal of Nursing **4:**240-244, 1903.
10. Goodnow, M.: Nursing history, ed. 9, Philadelphia, 1955, W. B. Saunders Co.
11. Information Service of India. Note on the history and development of the nursing services in India, 1977, unpublished manuscript. (Available from the Information Service of India, Embassy of India, Washington, D.C.)
12. Information Service of India. Nursing profession in India, 1953, unpublished manuscript. (Available from the Information Service of India, Embassy of India, Washington, D.C.)
13. John, K.: The advent of integrated health services in India, International Journal of Nursing Studies **2:**183-187, 1965.
14. Krishnan, S.: Planning nursing education for the 70s in India, International Nursing Review **18**(1):181-191, 1971.

15. Libbey, A.: Junior year in India, American Journal of Nursing **66:**332-334, 1966.
16. Macry, H.: Nursing in India, Hospital Progress **22:**283-287, 1941.
17. Marson, W.: India's project number one, Canadian Nurse **63:**45-49, 1967.
18. Paul, E. H.: Nursing program of the Indian Red Cross society, International Journal of Nursing Studies **4:**56-62, 1967.
19. Pé, A.: Hope for millions, Nursing Times **61:**1494-1495, 1965.
20. Saunby, D.: A candle-lighting service in Kolar, India, American Journal of Nursing **46:**873-874, 1946.
21. Subhadra, V.: An evaluation of public health services at an urban health center, International Journal of Nursing Studies **7:**257-265, 1970.

Chapter 19

JAPAN

The development of modern nursing in Japan has a different history. After the opening up of Japan to foreigners about 1853, German physicians drew many Japanese students to Germany, and the Japanese government also imported many German teachers to help in establishing hospitals and schools. The first hospital was built by the Government in 1857 and put in charge of a Dutch physician.[5] It is not surprising, then, that the early beginning and development of nursing in Japan was derived from the same system of German hospitals, and especially the German Red Cross system of training nurses.[4]

DEVELOPMENT OF MODERN NURSING

Under the auspices of the American Board of Missions, Dr. John Berry in 1885 established the first school of nursing for Japanese women, with Linda Richards in charge.[14] Three married women and two others were the first students. Miss Richards remained in charge for five years, but eventually the school passed into Japanese hands. Shortly after, another school was opened in Tokyo Charity Hospital by Dr. Takagi, a Japanese physician who studied in London and wanted, with the encouragement and approval of the Royal family, to introduce the Nightingale system.[4] In 1890 the Red Cross established a school of nursing in the Central Red Cross Hospital in Tokyo.[6] Ladies of nobility and of royal ancestry were encouraged to take the two-year course and thus to qualify as nurses. This was the Motherhouse system of Red Cross schools and hospitals, which was highly centralized and militarized.[2,4,8]

Another major development in nursing was the establishment of the great St. Luke's International Medical Center in Tokyo, accomplished through the combined efforts of the Protestant Episcopal Churches of America and the Japanese government. A school of nursing was founded in 1904 in connection with the center that later became the official college of nursing. The newly founded college had a three-year basic nursing course, followed by a year of postbasic education in teaching, supervision, and public health nursing. This four-year course that trained nurses for leadership positions was based on the curriculum organized by the National League of Nursing Education.[1,10] In 1928 the college of nursing was the first to be recognized and chartered by the Department of Education.[1]

NATIONAL NURSES' ASSOCIATION

Between 1917 and 1947, the educational requirement for admission to a nursing school was six years of elementary education plus two years of junior high school. During this period, graduates from the nursing schools earned certificates as nurses, midwives, or public health nurses. In 1948 the Public Health Nurse Midwife and Nurse Law was passed by the Ministry of Health and Welfare. It prescribed the qualifications, training, practice, registration requirements, and national examinations for both graduate nurses and assistant nurses.[13] At about the same time the national nurses' association, known as the Japanese Midwives, Clinical Nurses, and Public Health Nurses' Association, was registered by the Japanese government with the aim of promoting professional and general education.[10] As a result, the Red Cross Demonstration School of Nursing opened in Tokyo, to become a center for refresher courses for nurse administrators, nurse educators, and clinical nursing specialists.[8]

NURSING EDUCATION

Thus education of nurses changed with the changing qualifications, and educators came to realize that registered nurses must be able to understand how to deal with the needs of the people and patients with knowledge and techniques of the advanced medicine, hygiene, psychology, and sociology of modern times.[3] Under the 1948 law the length of education of nurses is three years after graduation from high school, or twelve years of general education. To be eligible for the national examinations for midwives or public health nurses, candidates must have more than six months of training in the respective areas in addition to their basic nursing education of three years.[9]

Also, with the enactment of the 1948 law, the assistant nurse, a new category of nursing personnel, was created. The assistant nurse under the law should practice nursing under the supervision of a physician, a dentist, or a registered nurse. The length of training of the assistant nurse is two years after graduation from junior high school, or nine years of general education. In 1951 provisions were made for an assistant nurse licensing system, which permits licensing by the prefectural governor after completion of the two-year program and passing the examination.[15]

To meet the increasing demands of the population, the government established a policy giving priority to quantity over quality of nursing personnel, strongly affecting the overall direction of nursing education. As a result, a large number of schools for assistant nurses have been established, presently exceeding the number of schools for fully qualified nurses. More schools are also being established that offer programs for assistant nurses, with more than three years of clinical experience, to make them eligible for the national examination for fully qualified nurses. A night

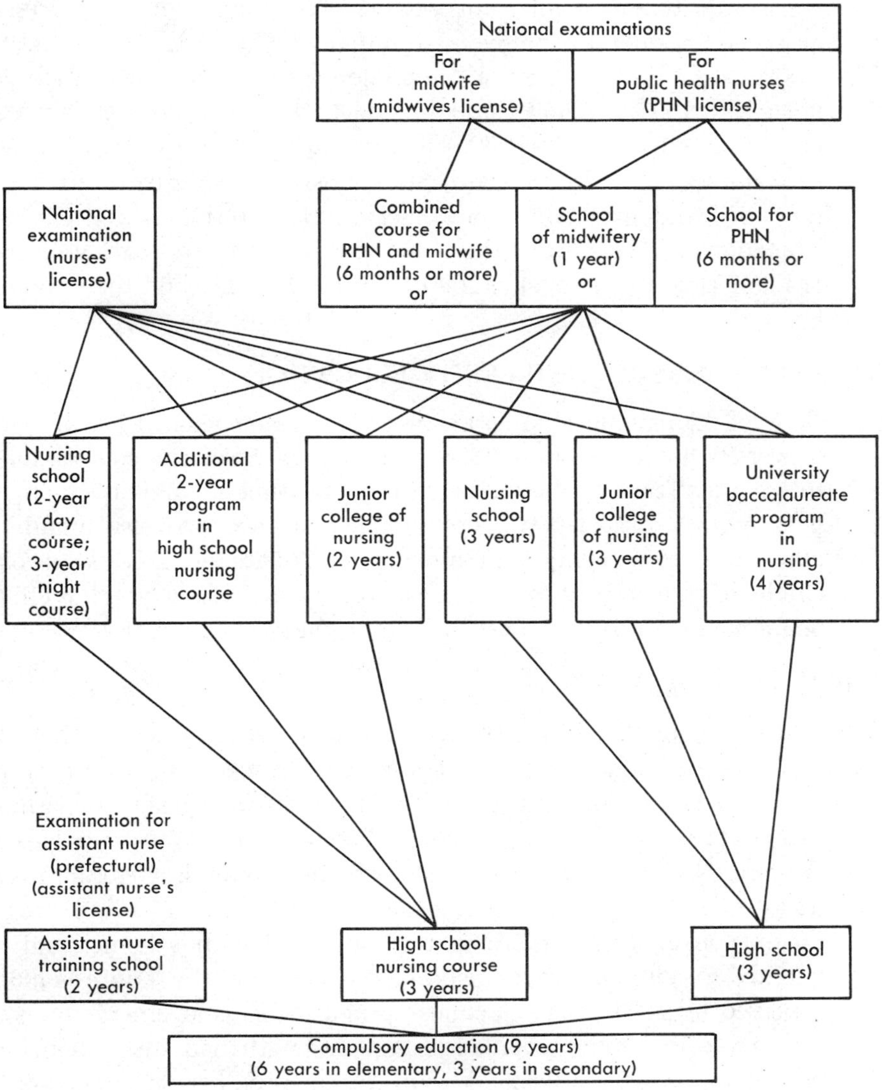

FIG. 12

Nursing education in Japan. (Modified from Tokyo Planning Committee, ICN Sixteenth Quadrennial Congress: Nursing education in Japan, International Nursing Review **23**(3):73-79, 1976.)

course is made available that was approved by the government for the training of assistant nurses. In 1964 another program was introduced by the Ministry of Education that involves a three-year vocational training course for assistant nurses at the high school level. Graduates of this program are allowed to enter the training program for assistant nurses to become fully registered nurses and hence obtain their nursing licensure. This makes the education system in Japan rather complicated, and as a consequence, many different ways of obtaining a nurse's license are available for students interested in nursing.[15] (See Fig. 12.)

After the development of comprehensive medical care, which was officiated in 1963, the government made an overall revision of the curricula of nursing education in 1969. The new curriculum was organized to prepare nurses who can provide comprehensive nursing care rather than to train the students mainly for clinical work in hospitals and clinics. The education of nurses under the new curriculum involves caring for patients or clients with due consideration for their daily life and their community living.[15]

ADVANCED NURSING UNIVERSITY EDUCATION

Baccalaureate-level programs were first developed in 1952. By 1975 ten university programs offered a nursing degree. Postbasic courses for nurse tutors are offered by the national local governments and also by the Japanese Nurses' Association. These courses are six to twelve months long; other short-term courses in nursing administration are also available.[15] Graduate education at the master's level is not available yet, but efforts are being made to institute these courses in the near future.[11]

PUBLIC HEALTH SERVICES

General public health services in Japan are provided at three levels: national, prefectural, and local government. Each prefectural government and local large municipal government has its own health department to carry out programs that are generally directed by the Ministry of Health and Welfare. National health insurance, which is compulsory for all residents, was established in 1938. In 1958 every city, town, and village was given the responsibility of enforcing the national health scheme, and consequently a comprehensive insurance system for the entire nation was achieved by 1961.[12] The Japanese primary care and emergency systems that cover the entire population have strengthened the national health program in making it available to every Japanese person in need of health care.[9]

Among the problems that Japan faces in the health field is the shortage of health facilities and manpower, including physicians and nurses.[7] Also, the fact that the typical nursing school or training institute is still of diploma level, in general sponsored by a private hospital, is a current problem for nursing education. Since most of the nursing is done by assistant nurses, a considerable effort is being expended in upgrading these programs, which are still dependent on medical associations. In addition, the country lacks continuing education programs for nurses who have been working for some time in clinical areas. Currently, the Japanese Nurses' Association is working on resolving these problems and on reforming the nursing education system, thus placing all nursing programs within the frame of higher education.

REFERENCES

1. Arak, I.: Nursing in Japan, American Journal of Nursing **28:**1003-1006, 1928.
2. Bullough, V., and Bullough, B.: The emergence of modern nursing, ed. 2, London, 1969, The Macmillan Co.
3. Chino, L.: Nursing in Japan, International Nursing Review **11:**19, Jan.-Feb., 1964.
4. Dock, L., and Stewart, I.: A short history of nursing, New York, 1938, G. P. Putnam's Sons.
5. Goodnow, M.: Nursing history, ed. 9, Philadelphia, 1955, W. B. Saunders Co.
6. Hayashi, S.: L'influence de Florence Nightingale sur le development des soins infirmières au Japon, Revue International de la Croix-Rouge **36:**272-278, 1954.
7. Iwasaki, H.: James Bond's nurse, American Journal of Nursing **68:**94-95, 1968.
8. Jameison, E., Sewall, M., and Suhrie, E.: Trends in nursing history, ed. 6, Philadelphia, 1966, W. B. Saunders Co.
9. Japan: health care for all and a demographic miracle, Hospital Practice **11:**157-158, 1976.
10. Jensen, D. M.: History and trends in professional nursing, St. Louis, 1955, The C. V. Mosby Co.
11. Kaneko, M.: A new aim of nursing education in Japan, International Journal of Nursing Studies **6:**141-149, 1969.
12. Kusakari, J.: Fact about public health nursing in Japan—changes during the years 1960-1970, International Journal of Nursing Studies **11:**3-19, 1974.
13. Nagano, S.: Nursing in Japan, Canadian Nurse **65:**35-36, 1974.
14. Richards, L.: Linda Richards in Japan, American Journal of Nursing **68:** 1716-1719, 1968.
15. Tokyo Planning Committee, ICN Sixteenth Quadrennial Congress: Nursing education in Japan, International Nursing Review **23**(3):73-79, 1976.

Chapter 20

CHINA

No record in Chinese history before the nineteenth century exists through which one can trace the words "nurse" or "nursing." In the past the care of the sick was mainly done by relatives and servants. In general, women were not educated, and those who could afford it were taught by private tutors. The teaching then involved the study of Confucian classics and the education of young girls to be obedient to their parents and husbands.[12] Around the middle of the nineteenth century, nursing care was provided entirely by a servant type of nurse who was trained to do some manual work, whereas medicine and treatment were entirely in the hands of the physician.[6,12]

BEGINNING OF MODERN NURSING

The first hospital was established in 1835 by Dr. Peter Parker of Canton, a distinguished missionary physician. Other mission hospitals were founded, but history records no attempt of their training nurses. The first graduate nurse to work in China was Elizabeth McKechnie Thompson from the United States, who went to Shanghai in 1884 to establish the first Nightingale system of nursing. British and Australian nurses trained under the same system also contributed to the development of modern nursing in China.[6,8,12]

With the turn of the century, education of Chinese women began bringing about the dissolution of old customs such as the foot binding of baby girls and the beliefs that women's place is only at home. Soon efforts were made to train Chinese women to become nurses. Male nurses were also trained, since it was thought to be improper for a woman to nurse a man who was not her husband—a belief that is presently waning.[8,11]

The first school for Chinese nurses was started by Ella Johnson in 1890 in a small mission hospital in Foochow. Practical nursing, midwifery, and dispensing were taught at the convenience of the teachers in a course that lasted two years. Other schools were opened, but none emphasized the educational background of the student. This opened the doors to the servant-type of nurse, since educated women were not yet willing to take up this task that was not highly esteemed by the public.[7,12]

NURSING DEVELOPMENTS

During the Russo-Japanese War in 1904, the Chinese Red Cross Society was established by Chinese residents in Shanghai. This was followed by the opening of a Red Cross Hospital in 1907 and a Red Cross School of Nursing in 1921. The Nurses' Association of China (NAC) was founded in 1909 by Cora Simpson, with the main purpose of establishing standards for nursing education and regulations for national examinations. By 1912 a standard curriculum was established, and a central committee was empowered to accredit schools. In 1915 the first examination for nurses was administered by the Nurses' Association of China, and in 1920 the first issue of the *Nursing Journal of China* was published. The Nurses' Association of China joined the International Council of Nurses in 1922 and has been an active member ever since.[11]

Many prominent schools were established in the same period, most of them under government auspices. The most notable one was the Nursing School of Peiping Union Medical College, which required senior middle school graduation but preferred college education. A combined university and nursing course was offered in affiliation with Yenching University. Graduates from this program held leadership positions in many parts of China, and some of them became leaders in hospitals and schools of nursing in the country. Although modern nursing and modern medicine were introduced into a number of cities in China, large territories of this country for a long time remained untouched and unapproached by these professions.[12]

Public health nursing, with all its possibilities for the elevation of living standards, was inaugurated at Peiping Union Medical College in 1925. The students of the school of nursing of the college, and students from other hospitals in Peking, affiliated with this program. Gertrude Hosmer organized the first public health nursing program in China. It comprised a nine-month postgraduate course, offered to graduates from the various Chinese schools of nursing. The Chinese government gradually developed this program by opening national schools of nursing throughout the country and making available scholarships to graduate nurses who were interested in working in public health.[10] Government involvement in the nursing profession was continuously increasing, and in 1937 the education of nurses was placed under the Ministry of Education. This change helped in the setting of standards for the registration of schools of nursing as well as the licensure of graduate nurses.[11]

HEALTH CARE IN COMMUNIST CHINA

During the eight long years of war, from 1937 to 1945, hospitals were established everywhere in China—in temples, factories, storehouses, mills, and schools—to compensate for the lack of transportation. Nurses worked under impossible conditions in meeting the war needs and in training aides and corpsmen. An army school of nursing was established in 1943, and nurses were given military rank. Help came to China from international organizations such as the Red Cross and the United Nations. Nursing activities during that period were hampered first by the war with Japan and later by the Chinese Communist regime, which reduced the educational standards of nursing by reducing the program to two years of training.[8,11] Most of the nursing schools were closed for the foreign nurses, and the missionaries in charge of them were labeled by the new government as agents of Imperialism and hence were expelled from the country.[2]

Since 1949, the year of the "liberation," the Chinese Communist government has made determined efforts to improve the health of the people by mass eradication of communicable and endemic diseases through the elimination of conditions that lead to these diseases and by health education of the public. This was made possible because the improvement of health care has been practiced by every segment of the medical community, including educational institutions, health facilities, and health practitioners at all levels. Major emphasis has been placed on the countryside, where the majority of the people live and where the medical facilities were the least available before 1949.[1,4,9]

HEALTH EDUCATION

Health education is widespread throughout China now, and medical training is available to everyone beyond high school. Villages and factories are supplied by health workers known as "barefoot doctors," who are commonly recruited from the area. Courses in health training are also available to every segment of the population, allowing graduates of one course to move easily to another. Many people in China learn a few basic acupuncture points and hence proceed to practice on themselves to perfect the technique that allows them later to become acupuncturists. The technique usually involves placing one or more needles in certain sites of the body and rotating them until analgesia is induced.[15]

Health education, in general, mixes theory with practice. Even schoolchildren of all ages spend a part of their academic year putting classroom theory into practice. Prospective nursing students in China are required to spend a period of time in the hospital as patient attendants and housekeepers before they enter a school of nursing.[1,3] Housewives, farmers, middle school graduates, and factory workers are chosen by the community to study for three or four months each year in their own local hospitals or health centers to become barefoot doctors and sanitarians; at the same time they are apprentices to physicians, nurses, midwives, acupuncturists, and dentists.[14] The barefoot doctors, after several years of part-time education and training, may be chosen to continue their education to be qualified to enter one of the other categories of health workers.[17]

Nurses, midwives, acupuncturists, physicians, herbalists, sanitarians, barefoot doctor, anesthetists, laboratory technicians, dentists, pharmacists, family planning workers, and medical and nursing students comprise the health workers' categories.[13] This provides for the existence of different levels of health workers but at the same time allows the easy mobility from one level to another. The beginners are usually people from neighborhoods or classrooms who are known as contact persons and who take the responsibility of checking to see that people in their area are receiving the proper medical care.[17]

Since the Great Proleteriat Cultural Revolution, the Peking Medical College has run an open-door schooling system by linking its educational revolution with the revolution in rural health work. Teachers and students of the college, led by the College Party Committee, did their best to reduce the shortage of physicians and nurses in rural areas. Courses were chosen to fit the needs of the rural areas and hence enable students to become professionals with a mastery of both Chinese traditional medicine and Western medicine, prevention and treatment of diseases, collection of medicinal herbs, and preparation of drugs.[5,16]

To raise the socialist consciousness and medical skills of the practicing barefoot doctors, a barefoot doctor college was established by the Nantung. Medical College. On completion of the course, students in the two-year program are required to retutn to the brigades from which they came and continue to work as barefoot doctors. Courses include lectures by physicians and political leaders of the community who coach students in their study of works by Marx, Lenin, and Chairman Mao.[16]

HEALTH CARE SYSTEM

To understand the Chinese health care system, one has to be familiar with the writings of Chairman Mao that provide the philosophical underpinnings of the whole system. Mao's concern, which has always been of the masses, is mainly reflected in the orientation of the health care providers. Mao placed the major emphasis of medical and health care on the rural areas—a not-surprising fact, since 80% of China's population live in rural areas. Fig. 13 will help the reader to understand the levels of health facilities as described by Chairman Mao. A Co-op Medical Care Plan at the brigade level ensures 100% medical enrollment of the population for a monthly premium of about 20 *fed,* the equivalent of 10 U.S. cents.[18]

Contrary to the widely held belief that the Chinese system is a fully sub-

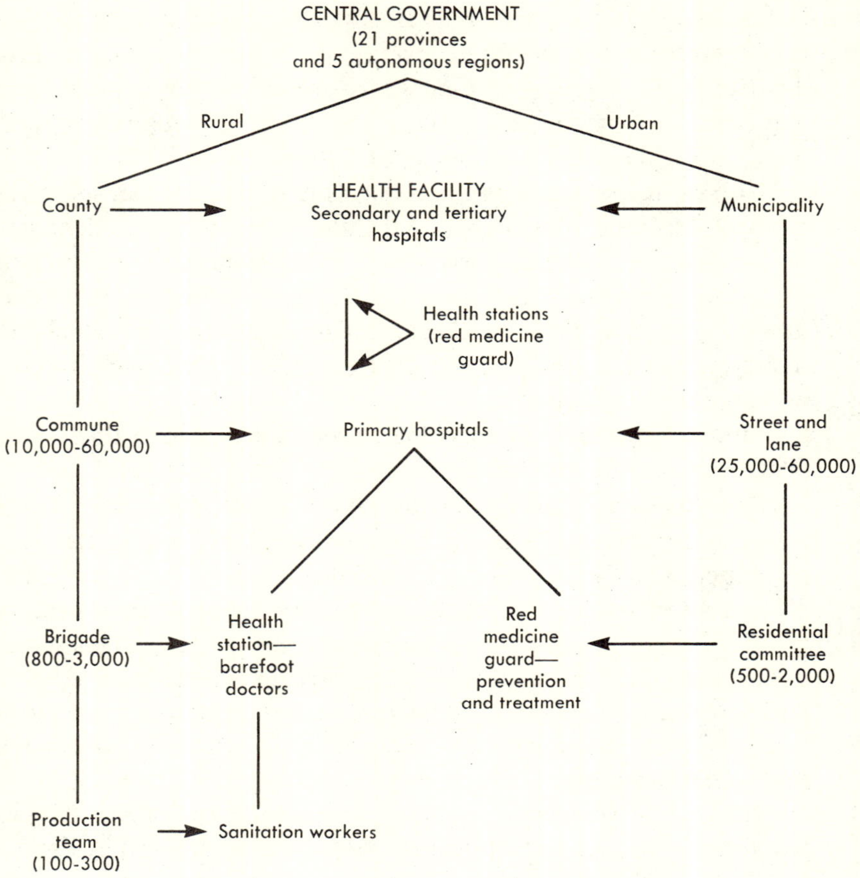

FIG. 13

Levels of health facilities in China. (Modified from Wen, C. P.: Health care financing in China, Medical Care **14**(3):241-254, 1976.)

sidized service from the government, a fee-for-service is the usual modality of payment for curative services in China. This is mainly because the government has delegated the operational responsibilities to the locality and region, which should be self-supporting and independent.

REFERENCES

1. Branch, M.: A black American nurse visits the People's Republic of China, Nursing Forum **12:**402-411, 1973.
2. Bullough, V., and Bullough, B.: The emergence of modern nursing, ed. 2, London, 1969, The Macmillan Co.
3. Chung, H. H.: An exploratory study of clinical nursing activities as a prelimi nary step for planning changes in care delivery system, International Nursing Review **18**(1):291-314, 1971.

4. Clawson, D. L.: When the green and the yellow do not meet, American Journal of Nursing **71:**1971-1973, 1971.
5. Deepening the revolution in medical education, Chinese Medical Journal **2**(2): 87-92, 1976.
6. Dock, L., and Stewart, I.: A short history of nursing, New York, 1938, G. P. Putnam's Sons.
7. Gage, N.: Stages of nursing in China, American Journal of Nursing **20:**115-121, 1919.
8. Goodnow, M.: Nursing history, ed. 9, Philadelphia, 1955, W. B. Saunders Co.
9. Gray, J.: East meets West in Canton, Nursing Mirror **142**(3):67-68, 1976.
10. Jameison, E., Sewall, M., and Suhrie, E.: Trends in nursing history, ed. 6, Philadelphia, 1966, W. B. Saunders Co.
11. Jensen, D. M.: History and trends in professional nursing, St. Louis, 1955, The C. V. Mosby Co.
12. Lin, E.: Nursing in China, American Journal of Nursing **38:**1-8, 1938.
13. Neonatal nurse practitioners, British Medical Journal **1:**115-116, 1975.
14. Pearson, S.: A peep behind the bamboo curtain: health services in China, Nursing Times **69:**243-244, 1972.
15. Revolution in health and education, Chinese Medical Journal **2**(2):149-154, 1976.
16. Stanley, M.: China: then and now, American Journal of Nursing **72:**2213-2218, 1972.
17. Wang, R. M.: China town in the classroom, American Journal of Nursing **74:** 113-114, 1974.
18. Wen, C. P.: Health care financing in China, Medical Care **14**(3):241-254, 1976.

Chapter 21

TAIWAN

Formosa, or Taiwan as it is known to the Chinese, is an island 85 miles off the southern coast of China, with a predominantly Chinese population.[2] During the period of Japanese occupation from 1896 to 1945, health facilities and nursing schools were limited, and those available were managed by physicians. Existing hospitals resembled hotels in which family members were allowed to stay with their patients and cook their food at the bedside.[4] Attitudes toward health care were inherited from Chinese traditions and Japanese medicine, which viewed nursing on a subvocational level. Under such a system the low level of esteem for nursing education at that time is understandable.[4]

DEVELOPMENTS IN THE HEALTH FIELD

Taiwan was a target for devastating bombing during World War II, leaving the hospitals and schools of nursing in poor condition. Within this framework and after the war, the government was faced with the problem of building adequate health facilities for the people and establishing educational programs to prepare nursing personnel. With the assistance of the World Health Organization and aid from the United States, some health programs, health centers, and stations were established. To meet the health demands of the country, nurses were needed, and an effort was made to develop nursing education. This was achieved through a survey carried out by the Nursing Department of the National Institute of Health in 1946. A direct outcome of the survey was the closure of hospital-operated schools of nursing, the establishment of a provincial school of nursing in Taipei for the training of nurse-midwives, and the initiation of refresher courses for hospital and clinic nurses.[4]

NURSING EDUCATION

In reconstructing Taiwan after 1946, the government followed the educational system that existed in mainland China, which was influenced by the British and American systems. Schools of nursing were established under two main categories: vocational and professional. Vocational nursing schools prepare nurses to function in hospitals and public health agencies. The three-year program requires students to be junior high school graduates with nine years of basic experience. The curriculum structure is based on the diploma programs, which give equal emphasis to theory and practice. These vocational schools, however, are limited to female, unmarried students under 22 years of age. Efforts are being exerted at present to recruit male students into these programs. At the completion of the programs, graduates are required to take the government examination to be licensed, which then allows them to take the title of "licensed vocational nurse.[4]"

Four-year baccalaureate programs and three-year college programs are also available to prepare professional nurses. Both programs require graduation from senior high school with 12 years of basic education. These programs are designed to prepare nurse teachers for the vocational schools and administrators for nursing service. The title of "licensed professional nurse" is given on successfully passing a higher level of examination. These graduates can go abroad for a master's degree, which entitles them to teach at the professional schools.[4] (See Table 1.)

In an attempt to upgrade the vocational schools of nursing, the government adopted the five-year nursing program proposed to the Department

TABLE 1
Nursing education in Taiwan*

	Type of training school							
	University or college of nursing		Junior college of nursing		Vocational nursing school		Technical colleges of nursing	
	Public	Private	Public	Private	Public	Private	Public	Private
Number of approved training schools	2	0	1	3	1	9	1	7
Length of training (years)	4	4	3	3	3	3	5	5
Entrance requirements	Female Senior high school No age limit		Female Senior high school No age limit		Female Junior high school Not more than 22 years		Female Junior high school Not more than 18 years	

* Modified from Educational system for nurses and midwives, Ministry of Health, Republic of China, 1975.

of Education in 1958. As a result, several nursing schools, named five-year technical colleges, are now in operation. These schools are designed to prepare clinical practitioners with a better foundation of clinical knowledge. Graduates can take either the vocational nurse or the professional nurse final examination, which allows the pursuit of graduate level education if the individual desires.

The nursing profession recognized the importance of preventive health care early enough to require all schools of nursing to include public health and public health nursing in their curricula. All nursing students also gain some public health experience through the hospital outpatient departments and the follow-up home care program. In addition, a twelve-month course in public health is made available by the Provincial Junior College of Nursing for graduate nurses who have had at least one year of public health experience. Scholarships are also available for graduate nurses who are interested in pursuing a public health specialists' degree in the United States, the United Kingdom, or Japan. This was accomplished because of the tremendous shortage of public health nurses in rural areas.[3]

MIDWIFERY

The practice of midwifery in Taiwan is governed by the Law for Midwives, which is set up by the government. Home birth and natural childbirth are much more popular than hospital birth in Taiwan. Midwives in private practice conduct the complete prenatal examination and are responsible for the pregnancy, birth, and postpartum periods. Midwives are presently prepared in many ways: a four-year bachelor's program, a three-year junior college program, a five-year nursing combined with midwifery program, a four-year nursing combined with midwifery program, a three-year nursing program, and a one-year midwifery program offered only to registered nurses. Midwifery as a profession is highly respected by society in Taiwan and hence attracts a large number of students.[1]

Nursing in Taiwan has gone through extensive changes in quality and quantity since independence. Within this period nurses have become university and college graduates, and nursing as a career has faced radical and rapid expansion in its structure, allowing it to provide more and better service to the society it serves.

HEALTH SERVICES

Public health services in Taiwan are administered at four governmental levels: national, provincial, county or city, and township. Each of these levels has its own health organization. The National Health Administration (NHA), established in 1971, is the highest authority at the national level. Under jurisdiction of the Executive Yuan, it determines health policies, formulates health programs, and supervises and coordinates health services at all levels. One provincial health department and one city health department are under direct supervision of NHA. They are responsible for the planning of public health and medical programs and the supervision of health activities of subordinate governments. Both public and private sectors render medical care services in Taiwan. The government provides free or subsidized medical services only to indigents; the rest of the population is responsible for financing its own medical care services.[5]

The Provincial Maternal and Child Health Institute was established in Taiwan in 1959. This institute, during recent years, has put into practice different projects that deal with maternal and child health services. Antenatal, postnatal, and child care clinics are the main activities of the maternal and child health stations that are scattered throughout the country. In addition, home visits are made regularly by the nursing staff, thus providing health supervision of the family as a whole. A considerable improvement in family planning education has occurred as the result of the intensive home visiting program of the public health nurses of the local health units. The Provincial Maternal and Child Health Institute is responsible for the training and supervision of the local MCH workers.[5]

The provincial health department has the overall responsibility of public health services in Taiwan, which include curative and preventive health services and in-service training of personnel. It is also responsible for supervision and planning of the county health bureaus and the health stations. The health bureaus are responsible for all the health services in their specific counties and cities. A health station usually serves a population of between 20,000 and 50,000. Its personnel comprise one or two physicians, two to five nurses and midwives, and one to four health workers.[5]

The National Health Administration of the Republic of China has developed a plan to construct more health facilities and to expand existing health stations to better serve the people of the area. Health education has played an important role in the improvement of the health care delivery system. Through health education the people have realized their own health needs and hence have cooperated with their own communities to strengthen the already existing health programs.

REFERENCES

1. Chang, C. T.: Maternity care in Free China, Bulletin of American College Nurse-Midwife **13:**139-142, 1968.
2. Jameison, E., Sewall, M., and Suhrie, E.: Trends in nursing history, ed. 6, Philadelphia, 1966, W. B. Saunders Co.
3. Li, S. F.: Public health nursing in Taiwan, Republic of China, American Journal of Public Health **56:**492-498, 1966.
4. Li, M. C.: The education and the role of the nurses in Taiwan, International Nursing Review **20:**176-177, Nov.-Dec., 1973.
5. Republic of China: Taiwan's health, 1974-1975, National Health Administration.

PART V

Africa

Chapter 22

SOUTH AFRICA

In the late 1800s, the South African Republic was sparsely populated with most people living on farms. Only when gold and diamonds were discovered were towns built and populated. This resulted in a thin distribution of medical practitioners all over the area. However, at that time most of the medical and all of the nursing care was done by the women of the household. The seasonal outbreak of malaria in 1878 and the annexation of South Africa to Britain, a move that precipitated the migration of many gold diggers, led to the opening of two emergency hospitals in the area. Women of the nearby villages, headed by a Mrs. Robins, took on the nursing of the malaria patients at these hospitals.[12]

EARLY NURSING DEVELOPMENTS

At about the same time, Sister Henrietta arrived in Africa from England to join the sisterhood of St. Michael and All Angels. Six years later she undertook to train nurses of the area who, until then, had been honorary helpers. Trained nurses were later sent to different parts of the country that had been stricken by epidemics of communicable diseases.[4] With the discovery of gold in South Africa, an economic boom resulted and public revenue increased rapidly. This brought about an increase of Dutch and English medical practitioners, who on their part pressed for more hospital facilities. All this contributed to a decision by the government to establish subsidized hospitals, causing an increase in the number of medical care facilities, the appointment of more medical consultants, and education of nurses in formal schools.[4,12]

Sister Henrietta's training methods included lectures by herself and by local physicians and surgeons on anatomy and physiology, practical nursing, and cooking. At the end of the first year of training, nurses were promoted to staff nurse but continued training for another year, at the completion of which an examination was taken. After a third year of training, nurses received a certificate that entitled them to be registered with the

British Nurses' Association. In 1891 South Africa was the first country in the world to pass registration laws for nurses.[8] This was attributed to the efforts of Sister Henrietta, who insisted that nurses should be given legal standing as properly qualified nurses, as distinct from volunteers. As a result, nurses were placed on the register of the Colonial Secretary's Office through the Medical, Dental, and Pharmacy Act.[12]

NURSING ORGANIZATIONS

On the termination of the South African War and the signing of the Peace Treaty of Verceniging, South African republics became British possessions. In 1910 the four colonies merged into a union of four provinces. A consolidating law was passed at the same time that controlled the practice of medical practitioners, dentists, chemists, druggists, nurses, and midwives. The first South African Trained Nurses' Association, founded in 1914, was represented by nurses and midwives on the South African Medical Council, which demonstrated an important example of physicians and nurses working together harmoniously and effectively.[3]

In 1944, in spite of many difficulties, a charter was granted by the government that established the first South African Nursing Council and the South African Nursing Association, replacing the South African Trained Nurses' Association. These two bodies together regulate the affairs of the nursing profession, the first being responsible for specifying the curricula, supervising the standards of nursing schools, and granting registration, and the second advising the Ministry of Health on nursing matters and working for the welfare of its members.[3,8]

NURSING EDUCATION

From 1900 to 1948, nursing and midwifery training was provided in a series of hospitals and nursing homes, ranging from private, profit-making, missionary institutions to state-subsidized institutions. An apprenticeship system existed at that time by which student nurses signed a contract with a hospital board to serve three and one-half years during their training period, leaving little scope for the development of a truly educational program.[3] Soon after World War II, the majority of nursing schools in South Africa were associated with a nursing college. Each nursing college was an educational center or teaching department that provided theoretical instruction for students from different hospitals and maintained close supervision of clinical practice. After three and one-half years in the basic nursing course and on passing the final examination, the student became a fully fledged registered nurse.[3,10]

To prepare nurses for community work or care other than at the hospital bedside, a basic degree program was developed in 1956 by the University of Pretoria. A Bachelor of Arts and a Bachelor of Science degree in nursing were established within the faculties of arts and sciences. Both programs were four and one-half years long, at the end of which graduates were registered as medical and surgical nurses. The training in both programs was patient centered, requiring nurses to be enrolled at the Pretoria Hospital as staff members. This was done mainly to emphasize the team concept early in the students' training and to develop responsibility from the start.[6] Candidates for both programs had to meet university admission requirements. The nursing content of the B.A. and the B.S. courses is the same. One, however, is weighted on the side of the social sciences, whereas the other focuses on the physical sciences in nursing.[9]

BANTU NURSES

Although the training of white nurses was expanding rapidly, Bantu women were still receiving on-the-job training as nurses' aides until the beginning of the twentieth century. This was attributed mainly to tribal prejudices, lack of sufficient high schools, the poverty of the people, and the tendency among the Bantu parents to give preference for education to their male children.[12] Training facilities for South Africa's Bantu girls are expanding rapidly. Training colleges for nurses with the same admission standards, requirements, syllabi, and examinations are being established throughout the Republic, and an increasing number of Bantu women are adopting nursing as a career. Because of the Republic's segregation laws, coloured Indian and Bantu cannot train with white people, and hence each group has its own colleges and training schools. General as well as postbasic nursing training is available in approximately twenty different courses, including nursing administration, clinical care, instruction, and midwifery programs.[2,5]

Although Bantu men had served as orderlies in nonwhite hospitals since 1856, no attempt was made to train them. However, in 1927 a course was introduced at the hospital to train male nurses to relieve female nurses on male wards.[5,7] Some Bantu male nurses were employed as health inspectors by the Department of Health to work in the Bantu Reserves or in the Indian townships.[12]

TRENDS IN NURSING EDUCATION

In addition to the aforementioned basic courses, two types of basic midwifery courses are presently available in the field. An eighteen-month course is offered to persons not qualified as medical and surgical nurses. The other is a nine-month course for registered nurses only. The standard of admission to the basic nursing school, which includes programs in psychiatric nursing, has been set at a minimum of ten years of general education.[13]

In 1966 the University of Pretoria, on the recommendation of the medical faculty, transferred the bachelor of arts nursing degree of the College of Medicine, thus establishing a Department of Nursing Science within this faculty. Six other universities soon established integrated baccalaureate nursing programs, two of them using English as the language of instruction and the others using Afrikaans.[1,11] However, all students use both languages in addition to a third foreign language. Also, unique to the university program in South Africa, of which nursing is an integral part, is the requirement of two majors for the degree, nursing being the second major.[1]

Postbasic education programs are also available in clinical nursing fields and in administration and teaching fields. Clinical training at present focuses on operating-room techniques, ophthalmological nursing, pediatric nursing, neuropsychiatric nursing, surgical nursing, orthopedic nursing, public health nursing, and occupational health nursing. These courses are administered at hospital schools of nursing or at technical colleges, depending on the nature of the course. Training in the administrative and teaching fields, available for ward sisters and clinical instructors, is usually conducted at the university level and extends for one to two years. Refresher courses for hospital nurses, offered also by local hospitals and schools of nursing, have contributed a great deal to the quality of nursing care given.[12,13]

In addition to the baccalaureate degrees in nursing, master's and doctoral degrees have been introduced at some universities in the country and are known as "Master Curationis" and "Doctor Curationis," referring to a special healing function that a nurse possesses. This has placed the nurse on a status in which full partnership is shared with the medical practitioner in the health care arena. Master's degree programs in nursing, available now in nursing education, nursing administration, and clinical nursing, have common core subjects with postgraduate medical students. The doctoral degree, however, is a research degree with in-depth study of two aspects of nursing.[1,11]

The curriculum of the baccalaureate degree extends for four and one-half to five years, and all universities require student nurses to be student members of the hospital and other health agencies where experience can be obtained. Ward staff share in the supervision of clinical experience; however, a major part of the clinical instruction is by the university personnel. A three-year baccalaureate program was introduced in 1970 by the University of Pretoria for registered nurses, with the purpose of assisting this group to meet modern nursing challenges. Other universities have since introduced such a program into their curricula, attracting many nurses who are willing to accept the challenges.[1,11]

REFERENCES

1. Bauman, M. B.: Baccalaureate nursing in a selected number of English speaking countries, International Nursing Review **19**(1):12-38, 1972.
2. Beal, B.: Bantu nursing, American Journal of Nursing **70:**547-550, 1970.
3. Bridges, D.: A journey to Africa, International Nursing Review **2:**7-13, April, 1955.
4. Bull, M. R.: Kimberly: a century of nursing, Nursing Mirror **133:**27-30, Dec. 17, 1971.
5. Bull, M. R.: Training South Africa's nurses, Nursing Mirror **133:**18-20, Dec. 24, 1971.
6. Erasmus, C.: Experiences of an exchange-visitor-nurse, International Nursing Review **14:**42-44, Aug., 1967.
7. Fendall, N. R.: The medical assistant in Africa, Journal of Tropical Medicine and Hygiene **71:**83-95, 1968.
8. Goodnow, M.: Nursing history, ed. 9, Philadelphia, 1955, W. B. Saunders Co.
9. Grobellaan, A.: South African experiments with the basic collegiate program, American Journal of Nursing **58:**1401-1402, 1958.
10. Roberts, E.: Nursing in Johannesburg, Nursing Mirror **129:**39-41, Sept. 19, 1969.
11. Searle, C.: Developments in nursing education at South African universities, International Journal of Nursing Studies **6:**107-113, 1969.
12. Searle, C.: The history of the development of nursing in South Africa, Cape Town, 1965, C. Struik (Pty) Ltd.
13. Searle, C.: Nursing education in South Africa, International Nursing Review **41:**49-62, 1957.

Chapter 23

NIGERIA

In Africa the presence of preventable diseases still is a major problem, and health standards are poor. Poverty, illiteracy, ignorance, poor sanitation, and lack of medical care contribute to the health problems. Hence, before attempting to treat disease, the social conditions that have caused it must be attacked. All these factors create a challenge for the provision of medical and nursing care in the developing countries. Since the number of physicians available is inadequate, many tasks that would otherwise be done by them are carried out by nurses or other paramedical personnel. In such a context one can find many interesting innovations with the use of health-related professionals occurring in most of the developing countries.[12,14]

Like other English-speaking countries among the developing nations, health services were organized in Nigeria at the turn of the present century. Originally, such services were meant for military men and their families and included European traders and missionaries. Gradually, the services were extended to the African population through the establishment of government clinics and hospitals. A sharp distinction existed between the curative and preventive services, with the government taking responsibility for cure and the local authorities for prevention. All physicians were trained overseas, since no medical schools were available in the country, explaining the scarcity of physicians at the time.[12]

DEVELOPMENT OF MODERN NURSING

Nursing in the sense of helping has a long and traditional history in Nigeria. Formal training of professional nurses was based on the British system and continues to the present time to dominate and influence the philosophy and curricula of most schools of nursing.[6] Apart from training obtained in Nigeria, many Nigerians went to the United Kingdom to undergo the three-year course there, followed by a year of either midwifery or public health.[11]

Registration of nurses and midwives in Nigeria started as early as 1910, but the Midwives' Board of Nigeria and the Nursing Council of Nigeria were not established until 1930 and 1946, respectively.[8] These two bodies, through the efforts of their leaders, have contributed a great deal to raising nursing standards throughout the country and to adapting nursing curricula to the people's needs.[12]

NURSING EDUCATION

At present, federal- and state-operated nursing schools are abundant throughout the country. All these schools are tuition free, and all qualify their graduates for registered nursing certificates that are recognized in Nigeria and throughout the United Kingdom. Generally, men are not encouraged to join the profession, although one all-male nursing school exists near Lagos. To be admitted to any one of the diploma schools, candidates should have the secondary school diploma and should be fluent in English in addition to the native language. A high score on the common entrance examination given by the Nursing Council is also required. The entire teaching scheme is patient centered, focusing not only on the care of the sick but also on the prevention of disease.[6]

In 1950 a midwifery school was established by British nurses that trained graduate nurses in a one-year program. At the end of training, students were permitted to take the examination set by the Nigerian Midwives' Board.[15] Similar schools were established to train domiciliary midwives in an effort to meet the country's needs for rural health services.[13] Under the same goals, health centers were built in rural villages, and community health nurses emerged whose training adapted well to the needs of the health center. Candidates for these programs are required to have had a minimum of nine years of general education before they are admitted to the three-year training, combining the essentials of midwifery, nursing, child care, and health visiting. Such programs are also made available to midwives, who are required to take a one and one-half year course before qualifying as community nurses. To assure proper and continuous health services, candidates are recruited from the rural areas. They remain in close touch with their own communities and thus are more likely to remain in those areas.[12]

Many children under 5 years of age were dying of infection, malnutrition, and ignorance. To meet these pediatric challenges, the child health nurse came into being. Nurses in the area make primary decisions, see and manage a large number of patients with uncomplicated illness, and refer the few complicated cases to physicians. This new role has expanded the functions of nurses in Nigeria and raised the standards of the profession in the country. The child health nurse is usually a registered nurse whose experience has been enhanced by a few additional courses on assessment and diagnosis of major and minor health problems. These functions are conducted in a clinic under the help and supervision of a physician.[10,12]

One year after Nigeria achieved full independence, the Federal Ministry of Health initiated official action that resulted later in the establishment of a postbasic nursing program at the University of Ibadan. With the help of the World Health Organization, a survey of the nursing conditions was conducted that made special reference to the lack of an adequate number of nursing schools and to the need of upgrading nursing education.[1] As a result of a joint effort among the World Health Organization, the Rockefeller Foundation, UNESCO, and the Nigerian government, the first Department of Nursing within the Faculty of Medicine was founded in 1964 at the University of Ibadan. The baccalaureate nursing program, which admitted its first students in 1965, is a three-year course focusing on the integration of theory and practice. The courses are specifically designed to prepare students to work in the areas of teaching, administration, or research in nursing. Throughout the curriculum, theory and practice are adapted to the needs of the indigenous locale and culture, thus rendering it more pertinent and useful.[4,7]

Because so many preventive aspects of health care are carried out by nursing personnel, all nursing curricula in Nigeria at all levels focus on this important part of the health care delivery system.[9] Some schools have devised a special postgraduate course in public health or community health nursing in an attempt to meet the growing needs of the population. In addition, most of these programs integrate prevention into all their nursing courses so that students will have a broad idea of what preventive medicine means and how positive health can be achieved. These nursing concepts help the nurses educate the public on the nature of disease and the different ways it can be prevented.[2,5]

NURSE TRAINING TODAY

For a student wishing to enter the nursing profession in Nigeria, four basic level programs are available as follows:

1. A three-and-a-half-year general nursing course is offered in schools of nursing attached to hospitals or University Teaching Hospital. This prepares the nurse to take the Nursing Council examination at the end of the program. Graduates who have completed the new standard of nurse education, introduced in 1965, are registered as "Registered Nurse (Nigeria)" or "(RN Nigeria)," whereas graduates of the old program are registered as *Nigerian Registered Nurse (NRN)*. However, both groups are designated as staff nurses on employment. The new program provides for general basic training, including courses in applied, general, and social sciences. This enables student nurses to choose their area of specialization early in their schooling.

2. A two-and-a-half-year course in midwifery is available at Maternity Hospitals Schools of Midwifery. On completion of the course the student is registered as "Nigeria Certified Midwife (NCM)" and carries the title of staff midwife on employment.
3. A three-and-a-half-year community nurse training course is also available. It is a comprehensive program in public health nursing. which includes health education and midwifery. Graduates of this course are registered as "Nigeria Registered Community Nurse (NRCN)" and also receive the midwifery certificate. Community nurses function in public health and preventive areas such as domiciliary health services, health centers, and infant welfare clinics.
4. A three-and-a-half-year training course in psychiatric nursing is offered at the Hospital for Nervous Diseases. On passing the qualifying examination, graduates of this course are registered as "Nigeria Registered Mental Nurse (NRMN)."[15]

The RN Nigeria graduate, after a few years of experience, can take postgraduate courses in teaching, administration, obstetrics, or research. However, most graduates take the one-year midwifery course. Nurses in this category who wish to go further can become health visitors by entering public health schools of nursing. The health visitor in Nigeria works with the family, teaching higher standards of health prevention.[3] The Bachelor of Science degree program at the University of Ibadan is another challenge for general trained nurses, providing opportunities for further study at the university level. Graduates of this program are prepared to serve as nurse educators or administrators in hospitals, schools of nursing, public health agencies, and similar institutions in the country.[15]

REFERENCES

1. Birch, J. A.: Nigeria in peace and war, International Journal of Nursing Studies **8:**145-152, 1971.
2. Bringing health to the nation, Occupational Health Nursing **22**(10):23-24, 1974.
3. Chokrieh, A. C.: Change in nursing in Nigeria, International Nursing Review **22**(3):71-79, 1975.
4. Clemence, B. A.: Baccalaureate nursing education in Nigeria, International Nursing Review **18**(1):40-48, 1971.
5. Davis, A. J.: Health problems and nursing practice in Sub-Saharan Africa, International Journal of Nursing Studies **12:**61-64, 1975.
6. Davitz, L. J.: Becoming a nurse in Nigeria, American Journal of Nursing **72:** 2026-2028, 1972.
7. Dosunmu, N. E.: Nursing as a career in Nigeria, International Nursing Review **20**(1):30, 1973.
8. Duke, E. O.: History of nursing in Nigeria, The Australian Nurses' Journal **65:**34-36, Feb., 1967.
9. Hamilton, J.: Nursing in northern Nigeria, Nursing Times **62:**259-260, 1966.

10. Mojekwu, V. I.: Pediatric education for Nigerian nurses, Journal of Tropical Pediatrics and Environmental Child Health (Kampala) **21**(1-B):72-73, 1975.
11. Muir, M.: Nursing in Nigeria, Nursing Times **63:**530-531, 1967.
12. Pratt, R.: The challenge of nursing in developing countries, International Nursing Review **17**(2):158-171, 1970.
13. Radwanski, D.: Occupational health services in Nigeria, International Nursing Review **19**(3):283-288, 1972.
14. Timmins, N. G.: Nursing against the odds, Nursing Times **61:**1763-1764, 1965.
15. Turtill, B. M.: Midwifery and midwife training in Nigeria, Nursing Times **61:** 1664-1665, 1965.

Chapter 24

MOROCCO

Morocco displays a blend of past civilizations that left only traces in the sand on their disappearance, and these traces make up today's Moroccan culture. Although Morocco is a Moslem-African country whose people speak and write Arabic, it is neither African nor typically Arabic or Moslem.[2] In spite of many obstacles, Morocco has made tremendous progress in developing health facilities to meet the needs of the country. The health center, which can be urban or rural, comprises the main unit of health services. Local dispensaries branch out of this health unit to serve subdivisions of the population. In these dispensaries nurses keep a continuous check on the health care of the community.[1]

NURSING EDUCATION

Nursing education in Morocco is under the Ministry of Public Health, which takes the responsibility in training and employing nurses. The Office of Professional Education, which directs and supervises schools of nursing, prepares both registered nurses and auxiliary health personnel. Out of twenty-eight schools responsible for the training of allied health personnel, one grants a postbasic degree in nursing, four grant the general nursing diploma, one offers a certificate in obstetrical nursing and one in neuropsychiatry, and fifteen train nursing auxiliaries.[1]

Candidates admitted to the diploma program in nursing must have six years of secondary education, be at least 18 years of age, and pass the entrance examination to the school. Auxiliary nursing students must pass an entrance examination and should have completed three of four years of secondary education. On completion of two years of practical experience, auxiliary nurses, if they desire to change their nursing status, are permitted to take the entrance examination of the schools for registered nurses as well as certain correspondence courses. On the other hand, registered nurses with one year of experience in nursing can take the entrance examination to the postbasic school of nursing in addition to some correspondence courses offered by the school.[1]

The two-year curriculum for registered nurses includes courses in general culture, social and human sciences, biological and physical sciences, pathology and nursing, and public health, including family planning. The postbasic program, also two years long, focuses on specialty courses in education, administration, social welfare, and obstetrical nursing, in addition to the advanced courses offered in the registered nurses' program. Auxiliary nurses are trained for nineteen months, during which theory and practice are integrated.[1,2] These programs are conducted by specialized instructors from the postbasic school or by registered nurses who went abroad for specialization. The curricula of the three types of nursing schools stress prevention and positive health. Since all Moroccan public health services are integrated, nurses at all levels, in urban or rural areas, are expected to participate in the prevention of communicable diseases, health education, maternal and child health care, and family planning.[1]

In light of the emphasis on continuing education for nurses to assure a better health care delivery system, the Ministry of Public Health has set up provincial and district committees to establish in-service and continuing education programs. These committees see to it that all nurses take part in the programs offered. The standard of care in hospitals is evaluated regularly by the Central Technical Services of the Ministry of Public Health, whose staff is composed of physicians and nurses who are competent in their areas. This ensures that proper health care is available to the general population.[1]

Noteworthy is the fact that 50% of Moroccan nurses are men, who consider nursing to be a worthwhile profession. Many of the male nurses, however, continue their education and become physicians.[2]

REFERENCES

1. Moutou, L.: A glimpse at the nursing profession in Morocco, International Nursing Review **22**(1):23-24, 1975.
2. Rogers, C.: Morocco: an exotic land, AORN Journal **21**:324-330, 1975.

Chapter 25

GHANA

EARLY NURSING DEVELOPMENTS

The care of the sick in Ghana was always carried out by elderly women in the community whose skill was acquired through experience in housekeeping and child rearing. Professional nursing dates from the colonization of the country by Britain in 1844. British physicians took care of the colonial administrators, and mission doctors worked among the pagans they were assisting to turn to Christ. Many male orderlies enlisted with the missionary groups to help bathe and feed the sick. Later, these orderlies were trained by physicians to dress wounds and administer simple drugs. Recruitment of female nurses for this type of work was impossible, since families regarded nursing as an unsuitable profession for young women.[3] Training in simple nursing tasks began in 1899 by a British colonial sister who organized an in-service program to train the orderlies, already in practice, for senior nursing posts that until then were mainly held by the colonial nursing sisters of Britain.[3]

NURSING EDUCATION

The first midwifery training school was established in 1928 in Accra, and high school students were recruited for midwifery training. On graduation the newly trained midwives assumed staff nursing positions in maternity hospitals or went into domiciliary midwifery. In 1931 the Midwives Board was established, which brought into force the legislation for the training, examination, registration, and practice of midwifery.[3]

In 1944 the first curriculum for the training of state registered nurses was established. The training of local girls followed the general standard practiced in England and Wales at the time. This made it possible for locally trained nurses to be registered in Britain. Another curriculum was drawn up during the same period for the training of candidates in mental health nursing. In addition, a public health nurse–training program was started to prepare nurse-midwives in a one-year postbasic course.[3]

NURSING LEGISLATION

The Nurses' Board of the Gold Coast and the Nurses' Ordinance were established in 1946 as a result of legislation introduced to govern the standard of training of state registered nurses, qualified registered mental nurses, and public health nurses and their examination, registration, and code of practice. As a result, examination and registration were done on a national basis, with the board supervising the practice of nursing and taking disciplinary action when deemed necessary. At present, three nursing divisions exist in the Ministry of Health in Ghana. One deals with nursing education, one with hospital nursing service, and one with public health nursing service. The head of the main division is the Chief Nursing Officer, who is assisted by the heads of the three subdivisions. The employment of nurses of all grades in the government service is done by the headquarter offices in Accra that plan the allocation of nurses according to need.[3]

HEALTH SERVICES

Health services are available at health posts in remote rural areas through health centers, district hospitals, regional hospitals, and central hospitals that offer all the specialist facilities. A typical health post serves a population of 10,000 to 15,000 and is usually staffed by a health post attendant, health inspector, community health nurses, and a midwife. Home visiting and preventive care are by the midwife and the community health nurses. The number of personnel, as well as the sophistication of their training, increases as one moves up the hierarchy in the health care delivery system. Patients are constantly referred from the health posts to the health centers for more specialized treatments and care.[6]

NURSING PERSONNEL AND THEIR TRAINING

Two categories of nursing presently exist in Ghana: a professional nurse, who is the state registered nurse, and the auxiliary nurse, who performs the less skilled nursing duties. The curriculum for the training of state registered nurses lasts for three years and includes psychiatric, public health, and obstetrical nursing in addition to the basic nursing courses. In 1963 a postbasic Department of Nursing was established at the University of Ghana at Legon for higher nursing education. This was made possible through a tripartite agreement of the World Health Organization, the government of Ghana, and UNICEF. Two-year programs are offered in nursing education and administration. Nurse tutors are prepared to teach general, psychiatric, and public health nursing and midwifery.[3]

Two categories exist in the training of auxiliary nurses: the enrolled nurses, or nursing assistants, who work in institutions, and the community health nurses, who are assistants to the public health nurses with special training in maternal and child health, who work in rural areas. Since the majority of problems in Ghana are categorized as public health problems, the Ghanaian public health nurse and the community nurse have proved to be extremely valuable in meeting the country's health needs.[2,3]

Public health nurses in Ghana are known as medicosocial workers, health teachers, and family advisors. They have knowledge of child care, social and welfare services in the community which qualifies them to assess the health needs of the family through home visits, and follow-up care. Since much of the health care falls on nursing personnel, all nursing curricula focus on prevention and positive health.[2,5]

In 1970, through the foresight of a group of physicians, the government embarked on a family planning program and a nurse-midwifery training school modeled after the program at Downstate Medical Center in New York City. The three-year course prepared midwives in family planning methods and implementation. Family planning nurses have done an extensive job of instructing women in rural areas on modes of contraception as well as performing the routine physical examination and tests for preventive measures.[1,4]

TRENDS IN NURSING

The preparation of nurses in Ghana is undergoing change continuously. Basic nursing curricula are being revised, and more postbasic programs are being added. In-service and continuing education are gaining in popularity to the extent that they are being enforced by the government. Nursing at the graduate level is becoming popular, and nurses are leaving the country for the United States to seek higher education in nursing. All these developments in nursing education, which have taken place over a short period of time, speak for the promises the nation holds for nursing care in the future.

REFERENCES

1. Addo, C.: The midwife in family planning Nursing Mirror **133:**34-35, Dec. 3, 1971.
2. Davis, A. J.: Health problems and nursing practice in Sub-Saharan Africa, International Journal of Nursing Studies **12:**61-64, 1975.
3. Kisseih, D.: Developments in nursing in Ghana, International Journal of Nursing Studies **5:**205-219, 1968.
4. Pendleton, E. M.: Ghana looks for the future, Bulletin of American College Nurse-Midwife **17:**78-81, 1972.
5. Swaffield, L.: Blending the best of both worlds—nursing in Ghana, Nursing Times **70:**1056, 1974.
6. Twumassi, P. A.: Scientific medicine—the Ghanian experience, International Journal of Nursing Studies **9:**63-75, 1972.

Chapter 26

EGYPT

Egypt is one of the most ancient and best known lands of the African continent. The innovation of a government program for the training of women medical aides was established early in the nineteenth century. It started as a rudimentary national health service and has continued to grow ever since. A School of Medicine was founded in 1827 to train Egyptian physicians. In 1832 medical instruction was extended to young women. This school was the first of its kind in the Middle East that trained women medical aides. At that time Egypt was still a medieval Moslem society where the role of women was mainly controlled by tradition and culture. However, with the outbreak of communicable diseases, women were needed to do community health work. This led a Dr. Clot in 1832 to establish a public health program and to train women to become *hakimas*, or physicians.[2]

THE HAKIMA SCHOOL

The school founded to instruct women medical aides in Egypt was referred to as the Midwifery School, since it emphasized obstetrics and infant care. The six-year course included much rudimentary theoretical science—an impressive amount of instruction for that period. Many obstacles faced Dr. Clot in his attempt to develop the program. Finding candidates was his major problem because Egyptian parents at the time did not allow their daughters to work outside the home. However, with time and endurance many young women became interested in the work other *hakimas* were doing and joined in.[2]

All students in the *hakimas* program, like other students in Egypt, were housed, fed, clothed, and instructed at the expense of the state. On graduation from the program, honor students were automatically appointed assistant instructors, whereas the others were assigned to duty in Cairo Civil Hospital and in health centers in various parts of the country. Generally, the *hakimas* remained in senior student status, without promotion in rank or advance in salary, until they were married. This heavy-handed paternalism on the part of the government threatened the existence of the *hakima* school, since few women were interested in leaving home for what they considered to be a menial occupation.[2]

The first step in broadening the school's activities occurred when the school for *hakimas* was annexed to the Civil Hospital in Cairo. There the *hakimas* were able to work with indigent patients at the outpatient clinics of the hospital. They also organized a team that was responsible for controlling communicable diseases through immunization and education. The *hakimas* and their school survived into the twentieth century and today continue to function in the Egyptian public health establishment. What the *hakimas* performed at that time of history is remarkable, especially since women and children were virtually inaccessible to physicians. The *hakimas'* training center was the only state school for women in the country.[2]

BEGINNING OF MODERN NURSING

In 1882 and under the British occupation of Egypt, professional nursing was introduced. It emphasized hospital training and was mainly dominated by Europeans. Egyptian women, with the exception of *hakimas*, remained at home and practically outside society in general.[2] One of the earliest schools in North Africa is attached to the large Kasr-el-Ainy Hospital in Cairo, which has attracted and trained a large number of nurses from the region. British matrons and sisters administered the hospital for many years. However, this responsibility was later transferred to Egyptian nurses.[3]

The Higher Institute of Nursing was established in Alexandria in 1955 with the assistance of the World Health Organization. With the objective of raising the health standards of the country, the Egyptian Ministry of Health and the medical faculty of the University of Alexandria cooperated with the World Health Organization to help establish the institute. The program leads to a baccalaureate degree in nursing, emphasizing public health and other aspects of nursing. At the beginning the teaching staff was provided by the World Health Organization. However, with time, and with the availability of fellowships and scholarships by the government and other international agencies, Egyptian girls were sent abroad for specialization. Eventually, these nurses assumed leadership roles in nursing schools and hospitals.[3]

NURSING EDUCATION

At present many schools of nursing offer the four-year baccalaureate program in nursing. A one-year internship in a clinical area is required after graduation from the program to consolidate experience before responsibilities are assumed. Another fairly recent program in Egypt is a course that brings nurse trainees and medical students together in joint sessions, reflecting the growing appreciation by the medical profession of what nursing is doing at present.[1] Many of these graduates have gone to the United States to seek graduate degrees at the master's and doctoral levels, and on their return to Egypt they have contributed in raising the standards of their profession.[1]

Some graduate programs in preventive health and nursing are offered at some universities in Cairo. Diploma nursing programs and auxiliary nursing programs still exist in large numbers in Egypt. Most of these schools follow a standard curriculum under the Ministry of Health. The Egyptian Nurses' Association became a member of the International Council of Nurses in 1961.[1,3]

REFERENCES

1. Bell, J.: Leadership and responsibility, Nursing Times **69:**1542-1543, 1973.
2. Kuhnke, L.: The doctoress on a donkey: women health officers in nineteenth century Egypt, Clio Medica (Oxford) **9**(3):193-205, 1974.
3. Stewart, I., and Austin, A.: A history of nursing, New York, 1962, G. P. Putnam's Sons.

Chapter 27

RHODESIA

Traditionally, nurse training in Rhodesia was mainly practical. Today, however, with increasing specialist demands on the medical profession, nurses are prepared to accept more responsibilities by acquiring more medical knowledge through theory and practice.[2] The first African students started to train as registered nurses in 1959. They were chosen for their ability to read and write and to understand the English language sufficiently to follow the three-year course without difficulties. Prior to that most nursing was done by missionary sisters and physicians who settled in Rhodesia late in the nineteenth century.[3]

NURSING EDUCATION

The training of nurses at present is modeled after the British system. This has ensured registration of graduate nurses in Britain and allowed for nurses to enroll in postgraduate courses, which are not available in Rhodesia. The training of male nurses for registration started in 1964, increasing in popularity ever since. Training programs are for three years and follow the same admission requirements and syllabus as that of the British system. However, the different diseases and social and cultural conditions common to the country take up a major portion of the schools' curricula.[2,3]

Student nurses spend the first eight weeks of training in the school in an introductory course covering subjects such as anatomy, physiology, first aid, physiotherapy, administration, and nutrition. Nursing theory and nursing practice are offered. Courses are planned following the block system of education, with students alternating classroom instruction with clinical experience. During the training period students return to the school for four other blocks of four weeks each and another two-week block to prepare them to take the state final examination.[2,3]

Midwifery and psychiatry training are also available in Rhodesia. Both courses are offered in two-year programs to graduate nurses and, like the general course of nursing, follow the British scheme of training. On graduation nurses are registered with the Medical Council of Rhodesia and with the Nursing Council in Britain.[2,3]

ADVANCED NURSING EDUCATION

Rhodesia, like other countries of the world that are aware of the need for different categories of personnel on the health team, has launched a program to train advanced clinical nurses to replace the medical practitioner in rural areas. This training is under the auspices of the Medical Council of Rhodesia, a statutory body concerned with education, registration, and discipline of the whole health team in the country. The two-year course, offered at Mpilo Central Hospital, is open to nurses who hold the general and midwifery training qualification and who have had at least two years of practical experience. The curriculum includes experience in community medicine, obstetrics, gynecology, neonatal care, family planning, anesthetics, clinical medicine, clinical surgery, and clinical pediatrics.[1]

On completion of the training course, the advanced clinical nurses are registered to practice by the Medical Council and are usually employed by the Ministry of Health. These nurses will assist a medical practitioner in running a hospital or staffing rural and district hospitals where medical practitioners are only available for consultation. Clinical nurse specialists are charged with the need to arrange suitable community medicine when working in isolated areas and hence cooperate with the community nurses, health educators, and health visitors to carry out preventive health programs.[1] This constitutes a step forward in the training of nurses in this African country, contributing to the development and recognition of nursing as a profession.

REFERENCES

1. Ross, W. F.: The advanced clinical nurse and the health team, Central African Journal of Medicine **21**:243-245, 1975.
2. Snelgrone, F. W.: A school to be proud of, International Nursing Review **21**:9-12, 1974.
3. Whitaker, B.: Mpilo Central Hospital, International Journal of Nursing Studies **3**:53-55, 1966.

Chapter 28

ALGERIA

Before independence, Algeria's medical and nursing services had been organized and staffed by the French, most of whom left the country after 1962. The seven years' revolt, from 1956 to 1962, caused complete chaos in Algeria. Hospitals and medical staff were attacked and medical supplies and equipment destroyed. After the war the Algerians were faced with the task of reorganizing health care services throughout the country. Because of the war, the lack of education for women, and prejudice against nursing as an occupation for women, nursing care was mainly performed by male nurses.[1,3]

The nationalization of private clinics took place in 1965, and all persons with some medical or nursing experience were mobilized as volunteers to help in rural areas. Efforts were also made to train nurses in the cities, chiefly in basic skills, so that they could assist in hospitals, clinics, and dispensaries.[1]

Along with local efforts that helped restore health services, the Algerians had a number of physicians who were sent by France as part of the French cooperation. In addition, the Comité Chrétian de Service en Algérie (CCSA), established in 1962, took responsibility for coordinating the aid (medical supplies) given by most of the world's Protestant churches. Medical services, also provided by this organization, involved the opening of clinics and dispensaries and the training of paramedical workers, who later carried on the work previously done by the foreign medical staff.[1]

HEALTH EDUCATION SERVICES

Paramedical centers provided the following three grades of training:

1. An eleven-month course trained students to become midwives, nursing aides, laboratory and x-ray technicians, and children's nursing assistants.
2. A two-year program prepared male students to become nurses and laboratory assistants and female students to become midwives and *assistante sociale,* or social workers.

3. A three-year curriculum prepared students to become sanitary inspectors and eventually to take charge of clinics and dispensaries in rural areas.[1,2]

Since 1965 new hospitals have increasingly been built in Algeria. Almost all the population now receives free medical care through dispensaries, clinics, and hospitals that constitute the unit of health service in different districts of the country. Paramedical schools, administered by the Ministry of Health, train general nurses, pediatric nurses, rural midwives, physiotherapists, and dietitians in a two-year program. Several of these centers are now available in Algeria. Students qualifying for the programs become civil servants, since they are confronted with an enormous job for which they dedicate their lives.[1,2]

REFERENCES

1. Bull, M. R.: Health services in Algeria: the formation of a new service for a new country, Nursing Mirror **128:**31-33, Jan. 10, 1969.
2. Cowen, E.: Algeria—public health in an emergent state, Nursing Mirror **136:**33-35, March 16, 1973.
3. Stewart, I., and Austin, A.: A history of nursing, New York, 1962, G. P. Putnam's Sons.

Chapter 29

ETHIOPIA

The first medical or nursing personnel trained in Ethiopia were known as *dressers*. Training programs, established in 1948 and 1949, with the assistance of the World Health Organization Field Mission, provided hospitals and rural areas with personnel who had some kind of nursing knowledge. Male students with limited schooling were the only participants in the six-month courses. At the end of the training period, certificates were presented by the Emperor himself in a graduation ceremony. Some of the more capable students were encouraged after a few years of clinical experience to take another six-month course in nursing or to take specialized courses in x-ray or laboratory technology, pharmacy, or operating room techniques.[1,2] Throughout this period foreign nurses from different parts of the world administered nursing care in the country.

MODERN NURSING IN ETHIOPIA

In 1949 the first nursing school was established by the Red Cross Society in Addis Ababa with a Swedish nurse in charge. Another school soon followed, known as the Princess Zauditu Memorial School of Nursing, which functioned under the auspices of the American Seventh-Day Adventist mission. A school for male nurses was also opened at the Tafari Nokonen Hospital. In 1951 the Princess Tsahais Memorial Hospital and School of Nursing were established in memory of Princess Tsahais, daughter of the Emperor Haile Selassie. The emperor and empress were interested in nursing and hospital work, possibly because their daughter showed interest in the profession by seeking training in England during World War II. However, on her return to Ethiopia she died in childbirth.[2]

The programs in these schools last for three and one-half to four years and are under the supervision of the Medical Education Board, established by the Ministry of Health. Directors of the schools of nursing are members of the board and hence endeavor to standardize programs in the schools—a step that contributed greatly to the development of the nursing profession in Ethiopia.[2,4]

The Ethiopian Nurses' Association was admitted to the International Council of Nurses in 1957.[3] This and other developments are promising indications that nursing has wisely combined features of different existing systems and adapted them to the needs of the people.

REFERENCES

1. Goodman, M.: Nursing and the WHO, American Journal of Nursing **49:**134-136, 1949.
2. Magnussen, E.: Nursing in Ethiopia, American Journal of Nursing **53:**296-297, 1953.
3. Stewart, I., and Austin, A.: A history of nursing, New York, 1962, G. P. Putnam's Sons.
4. Wooldridge, R.: Nursing in a famine, Nursing Times **72:**166-167, 1976.

PART VI

South Pacific

Chapter 30

AUSTRALIA

Nursing in Australia goes back to 1838, when a group of Irish nuns arrived in New South Wales to found St. Vincent's Hospital. They were followed in 1868 by the first trained nurses sent from England by Florence Nightingale to work in Sydney Hospital, established in 1788. Lucy Osburn, the Lady Superintendent, had the entire responsibility of the nursing staff, composed mainly of nurses and wardsmen, and of the establishment of the training school for nurses. Women were engaged in the school as probationary nurses or sisters, whereas male nurses worked in male wards. This plan met with opposition from the medical staff, who disapproved of the employment of women as nurses and hence gave them little support. However, this opposition diminished with time to give way to the development of training schools throughout the country.[5]

Private nursing was the main field for some graduates, who shared living accommodations in nurses' clubs or cooperatives. However, in 1885 associations for district nurses were developed in most cities, allowing nurses some freedom in arranging their work schedule.[8]

NURSING ORGANIZATIONS

The first attempts at organization of the nursing profession in Australia were made in 1898 by a group of New South Wales nurses who decided to establish some sort of control of nursing and nurse training. This movement resulted in the creation of the Australian Trained Nurses' Association in 1899. It was followed two years later by the formation of the Victorian Trained Nurses' Association. Membership in these organizations was required of all nurses who were seeking a nursing post. The main objective of the nurses' associations was the establishment of a system for nurse registration in the whole country. *The Australasian Nursing Journal*, started in 1903 as the official organ of the Australian Trained Nurses' Association, became one of the world's oldest nursing journals. This was followed by *Una,* a journal adopted by the Victorian Trained Nurses' Association.[1]

Although efforts for state registration were made as early as 1909, only in 1927 did all states adopt it. The Nurses' Ordinance, which operated in the commonwealth territory, was passed in 1933. In addition to the ordinance, Nurses' and Midwives' Acts were passed in each of the six states of the Commonwealth, allowing a registered nurse in one state to be eligible for admission to the registers of the other states. Registration was granted to nurses trained in an approved school and examined by a recognized body of examiners.[5]

Each of the six states has its own professional organization. However, the state organizations are loosely knit into the Australian Nursing Federation, which is affiliated with the International Council of Nurses. The federation has helped to standardize the training of nurses throughout Australia as well as the development of postgraduate nursing programs. The federation now represents the whole organized body of nurses throughout Australia and is the recognized national association of all nurses in the country.[3]

DISTRICT NURSING

In 1909 an appeal was launched by the Countess of Derby, wife of the Governor General of Australia, to found a bush nursing service to supply nurses to the more isolated areas of the country. This was met with great opposition by physicians and nurses, and hence the service did not materialize. The Countess then turned to Amy Hughes, General Superintendent of the Queen Victoria Jubilee Institute, to organize an order of nurses in Australia similar to England's Metropolitan District Nurses. Today the Victorian Bush Nursing Association has many bush nursing hospitals and nursing centers throughout the country. Hospitals that were once isolated in small communities have served the large towns that have grown around them ever since. Nursing practices in these hospitals are patterned on the British system. However, most bush hospitals are established and controlled by the local communities. Apart from making medical decisions, nurses in the bush nursing centers carry a heavy responsibility, at times being miles away from the nearest physician or a larger medical center.[2]

Another voluntary organization that provided nursing service for the hinterland and the nearby Pacific islands was the Australian Inland Mission. Services of nurses in this mission are world renowned. An example is the work done by Sister Elizabeth Kenny, whose isolation in a doctorless area led her to the discovery of a new method for the treatment of poliomyelitis. The flying doctors, who now serve the "outback," tend to strengthen these nursing posts. Hospital planes and wireless stations make it possible for settlers in remote areas to get free medical consultation and the services of physicians and nurses needed.[8,10]

NURSING EDUCATION

Through Australian history the nurse has been seen as a health worker who requires a different kind of education from other members of the health team. The hospital-based apprenticeship system persisted in nursing for a long time while other health workers developed different kinds of institutions. Since nurse training was in the form of an apprenticeship, the socialization of nursing students started with conformity to hospital regulations and organization. Such a system that called for low entrance requirements and live-in accommodations provided the community with nursing service at a low cost. In addition, discipline is still emphasized as a major yardstick in the training of nurses in Australia. This is criticized by nurse professionals, who think the situation hampers development of the profession.

In spite of the fact that university nursing programs developed in North America and other parts of the world, the apprenticeship system of nurse training has survived in England and Australia. For a long time in England the traditional structure of the university refused to admit such a specialized and practical department as a nursing school to its campus. To hamper any further developments in the profession, nursing education in Australia was excluded from tertiary institutions as well. This was attributed to the inability of the profession to describe its own role in the health field at the time. To illustrate this better, the sociologist Hans Mauksch used the analogy of a flattened sheet of biscuit dough in describing the inheritance of nursing. In his opinion many new specialized personnel on the health team cut biscuits in terms of their specialized services to the patients. These people include technicians, therapists, social workers, and pharmacists, who staked their claims in patient care, leaving nursing with pieces of disconnected scraps of what was once the whole sheet of dough. More biscuit cutting continues, which leaves the nursing profession in the position of coordinating the pieces—the functions—to get the various services to the patient.[4]

Nursing educators recognized the importance of upgrading nursing education. As a result, the College of Nursing in Australia was established in 1950, with its first courses conducted in Melbourne, New South Wales. Subsequently, branches were established in other parts of the country. The college offers full-time postgraduate courses in nursing education, nursing administration, hospital nursing and ward management, public health nursing, operating room nursing and management, and intensive care nursing and management. The courses, varying in length from twenty-eight to forty-two weeks, are offered to hospital nurse graduates who are interested in a specialty area.[4]

In 1974 a diploma nursing course was started at the College of Nursing, leading to state registration under the general nurse category. This program will have wide implications in Australia, since it has the potential of changing the apprenticeship system of nursing education.

The nursing organizations are struggling with government authorities to improve the status of the nursing profession in their country. The Australian Trained Nurses' Association, known today as the Royal Australian Nursing Federation, with branches in all the states and mainland territories, is concerned with regulating the quality of nursing practice and nursing education. Only hospitals that conformed to the regulations set by the federation were recognized as nursing schools and their graduates allowed to register as trained nurses with the federation. This measure has helped to protect the trained nurses and the public against untrained personnel in the nursing field.[4]

COLLEGES OF ADVANCED NURSING EDUCATION

In 1964 the report of the Committee on the Future of Tertiary Education in Australia, known as the *Martin Report,* emphasized the need for the future development and diversification of tertiary education in the country. The focus was on Colleges of Advanced Education that share the same university status; however, emphasis is more on a practical than theoretical approach to education. This scheme was supported by the Commonwealth government that assisted the states financially in their efforts to establish the different Colleges of Advanced Education. The Victoria Institute of Colleges Act, passed by the government in 1965, was followed by the establishment of an Institute of Colleges in Victoria. The newly funded institute acts as a coordinating agency with which individual Colleges of Advanced Education may become affiliated.[6]

The New South Wales government, on the other hand, devised its own legislation plan for advanced education—the New South Wales Higher Education Act of 1969. The legislation provides for the establishment of a board instead of an institute, whose responsibility lies in the promotion, encouragement, development, improvement, and maintenance of advanced education courses. In 1972 the Council of the New South Wales College of Nursing decided that the college should become a school of nursing within the paramedical college, which comprised the colleges of physiotherapy, occupational therapy, speech therapy, and postgraduate nursing education.[6] This change has marked a sharp distinction between the New South Wales Colleges of Nursing and the College of Nursing in Australia, which is a single-purpose College of Advanced Education. The Commonwealth appears to favor creation of larger multipurpose Colleges of Advanced Education, as is the case in the Institute of Paramedical Studies.

GOALS IN NURSING EDUCATION

The changing pattern of health care needs and delivery, together with the rapid expansion in scientific knowledge, demands a change in the nursing education system. The nursing profession was presumed to be unable to provide adequate services to meet community needs in Australia. The nursing profession, at present, believes that nursing education should be phased into the general education system and the nursing programs placed at the tertiary diploma level. That graduates of these programs be competent and safe nursing practitioners is the concern expressed by the nursing leaders of the country, who speak for the goals of nursing education in general.[7]

Two categories of nursing personnel are presently functioning in Australia—the professional nurse and the auxiliary nurse. The educational programs that prepare professional nurses are conducted by the multidiscipline education institutions at the tertiary diploma level, whereas those which prepare auxiliary nurses are conducted by multidiscipline education institutions at the subtertiary level. The main goal is to establish basic nursing programs for professional nurses that provide learning experiences with students of other fields in the health professions. Such programs are intended to contribute to the promotion of effective functioning of the health team.[7]

The development of postbasic programs in nursing is a new trend in nursing education in Australia. These programs are designed for professional nurses who are graduates of either the hospital-based programs or programs conducted by multidiscipline education institutions. Appropriate bridging courses are made available to hospital graduates to help them gain entry into the postgraduate diploma or degree programs. Continuing education is also available to nurses employed in hospitals and health agencies to keep them up to date on new developments in the health field.[7]

ROLE OF THE NURSE

At present the nurse's role in Australia is accepted as complementary to that of the physician. In addition to providing general physical care, the nurse is viewed as a healer, advisor, comforter, confidante, and technician. The nurse is accepted by the public as a person on the health team who can advise on physical and mental health promotion, prevention of disease, treatment, and rehabilitation. As a primary health worker, the nurse is the first person whom the patient contacts, and consequently the proper delivery of care in the health system depends on the nurse's judgement.[9]

Australian nurses function in many capacities. In the hospital their activities vary from basic physical care to complex technical procedures. In the nursing homes, activation and rehabilitation of the patient are their main concerns. In the district nursing services they focus on the whole family. Nurses in child health centers are responsible for routine physical examinations and are actively engaged in the prevention of disease through the proper education of parents. The bush nurses in most instances have to act without medical assistance. Thus in some situations they have to take complete responsibility for diagnosing, doing minor surgery, deciding on drug administration, and caring for obstetrical patients.[9]

The community, or public health, nurse fulfills an expanded version of the role of the nurse, known elsewhere as the health visitor, whose emergence resulted from the need for a general nurse to support the general medical practitioner. The functions of a trained community nurse include (1) provision of services to families at home or at a neighboring center, (2) nursing treatment at home, (3) follow-up of patients referred from other centers, (4) referral of problems to the general practitioner physician, and (5) mobilization and coordination of services required by patients.[9]

Centers for group practice constitute the primary health facilities in Australia. A center is established close to a health department that coordinates neighborhood programs. The group practice employs a practice nurse, a receptionist, and secretarial help. The neighborhood health program utilizes community nurses, a medical officer, and social workers. The community nurse is the single point of contact between general practitioner and patient, mobilizing curative and preventive services. The nurse in Australia acts in an expanded role as a bridge between patient and physician. The final responsibility of patient care, both legally and morally, lies in the hands of the general practitioner.[9]

HEALTH SERVICES

Health services in Australia at the turn of the century were voluntary organizations supplemented by government subsidies and patients' fees. With the emergence of new techniques, hospital equipment became more expensive, leading to an escalation in the cost of medical care. The government had to intervene, accepting more responsibility in administering and financing hospital services. In 1945 the Chifley government introduced free public hospital treatment—a scheme achieved through agreements between the Commonwealth and the various state governments. The Commonwealth compensated the governments by paying 6 shillings a day for each occupied bed. Under the Hospital Benefits Act of 1951, the Menzies government approved a new agreement based on voluntary hospital insurance against costs of hospital treatment. The Commonwealth government paid 8 shillings a day for each occupied bed, and additional payments were made to patients who were members of a registered hospital benefit organization. With the exception of the Queensland Labor government, which refused to reintroduce charges for public hospital treatment, other states received a subsidy of 20 shillings a day until 1969, when sections of the Health Insurance Act were implemented.[4]

Alterations in the financing of medical services are being debated. A universal health insurance scheme has been proposed by the commonwealth government, entitling all citizens to standard ward hospital treatment and coverage against medical expenses at no charge. Health care is introduced on the premise that it is a right and not merely a personal responsibility. The organized medical profession constitutes the principal base of opposition to this scheme. Nurses, despite their numerical importance in the health care delivery system in Australia, have remained detached from the situation.[4] This reluctance of nurses to become involved in controversial issues is attributed to their acceptance of medical authority in the health field. If nursing is to grow as an independent profession, nurses must engage in debates on issues concerning their welfare and the welfare of the patient and the community.

REFERENCES

1. Bell, J.: Nursing conditions and problems in Australia, International Nursing Review **1:**123-127, 1926.
2. Boorer, D.: Nursing in Australia, Nursing Times **70:**844-845, 1974.
3. Burbridge, G.: Nursing in Australia, American Journal of Nursing **48:**226-228, 1948.
4. Dickenson, M., and Law, G.: Nurses in the national health scheme, Lamp **33**(3):30-36, 1976.
5. Evans, E. P.: Nursing in Australia, International Nursing Review **12:**260-264, 1938.
6. Parsons, R.: Trends in nursing education in colleges of advanced education, Lamp **30**(6):6-32, 1975.
7. Royal Australian Nursing Federation: Goals in nursing education, Australian Nurses' Journal **5**(10):11-14, 1976.
8. Stewart, I., and Austin, A.: A history of nursing, New York, 1962, G. P. Putnam's Sons.
9. White, R.: The role of the nurse in Australia, Canberra, Australia, 1972, National Health and Medical Research Council.
10. Wyndham, O. H.: Royal flying doctor service of Australia, International Journal of Nursing Studies **7:**39-53, 1970.

Chapter 31

NEW ZEALAND

The first nurses who trained under the Nightingale system went to New Zealand in 1883 and helped inaugurate a form of nursing training for upper middle class women. The apprenticeship system was adopted, and most nursing schools were parts of public general hospitals. By 1889 schools of nursing had been organized in three cities, Wellington, Auckland, and Christchurch, and soon their graduates introduced this new system of nurse training into other parts of the country. The school, hospital, and staff had to be approved by the Nurses' and Midwives' Registration Board and were continuously inspected by the Department of Health. Nursing and domestic services at the hospital and the training of nurses were the responsibility of the lady superintendent of each hospital. As a result, the matrons held a strong position in the country and became the nursing leaders in the large centers.[2,10]

The Nurses' and Midwives' Registration Board established regulations for nursing education that had little emphasis on theoretical instruction. The practical experience of the students covered medical, surgical, and communicable disease nursing, pediatric nursing, operating room techniques, outpatient services, and dietetics. Obstetrical nursing was never a basic course; it was offered at the postgraduate level only. A state examination was held at the end of the first and third years of the three-year basic nursing program. The final examination covered written as well as practical nursing subjects. Nursing education in New Zealand was free, and student nurses received a monthly stipend in return for their service in the general hospital.[2]

GOVERNMENT REGULATION

The Nurses' Registration Act, drafted by Grace Neill, who was the Assistant Inspector of Hospitals, became law in 1901. The Midwives' Bill was passed in 1904, providing for the training of midwives in state obstetrical hospitals. The training took place in state-aided schools, which were under the direct supervision of Grace Neill and later her successor, Hester Mclean, who helped direct the national program for maternal and child health in New Zealand.[2,10]

In 1906 a nationwide voluntary organization was started that greatly influenced the establishment of child health care in New Zealand. The Royal New Zealand Society for the Health of Women and Children was formed to help sponsor Dr. Truby King's child care program. At present, this society is called the Plunket Society, after its patroness Lady Plunket, wife of the then Governor General. Local branches were soon developed in different parts of the country known as Plunket clinics, in which specially trained nurses taught mothers the care and feeding of their babies. The Plunket Society also established Karitane Hospitals for babies needing special care and for the training of Karitane nurses. However, these hospitals were closed in 1977, and neonatal nursing care is now provided in intensive care nurseries in general hospitals. Attracted by the society's work, the government passed the Child Welfare Act in 1906, marking the beginning of a broader responsibility in this area.[10]

The Division of Hospitals and the Division of Nursing were formed in the Department of Health in 1920. The Division of Hospitals fell under the direction of a medical practitioner, whereas the Division of Nursing was the responsibility of a registered nurse and a midwife. The Division of Nursing was responsible for the supervision of training, examination, and registration of nurses, maternity nurses, and midwives; for the supervision of public hospitals and training schools and of district nursing services; and for the establishment of postgraduate courses in nursing. The Nurses and Registration Act of 1925 governed the registration of nurses, maternity nurses, and midwives.[2]

NURSING ORGANIZATIONS

New Zealand had many private nurses' associations as early as 1905. The first steps toward a national nursing organization were taken by Hester Mclean when she called on the separate associations to join together in one national association. As a result, the New Zealand Trained Nurses' Association, known now as the New Zealand Registered Nurses' Association, came into being in 1909. Midwives, maternity nurses, and some physicians were among its active members, in addition to registered nurses. The association became a member of the International Council of Nurses in 1912. *Kai Tiaki* became the association's nursing journal in 1923 and was edited by Hester Mclean, who founded the journal in 1908.[2]

The New Zealand Registered Nurses' Association has many branches scattered throughout the country. In addition to a matron's section, two others are devoted to public health nursing and nursing education. An affiliated student nurses' association, formed of the different councils representing the schools of nursing in the country, constitutes a section in the association. The student nurses' section of the main association was especially active in raising scholarships for study abroad.[10]

NURSING COUNCIL OF NEW ZEALAND

The Nursing Council of New Zealand was constituted under the Nurses' Act of 1971. The council is responsible for the nursing education programs, examination, and registration of nurses. The selection of curriculum content by the council is based on the principle that all subject matter should be integrated and applied to the total nursing care of the patient. In addition, the council undertakes the responsibility of conducting an ongoing evaluation program of all technical institutes and schools of nursing at all levels. One of the council's main duties is the formation and maintenance of the register, a challenge that the council has managed to handle ever since its development.[8]

NURSING EDUCATION

Nursing education in New Zealand since its early days had a tendency to follow the British system. This tie was strengthened during World War II, when many nurses from New Zealand served in Britain and often remained for postbasic education. Many British tutors were also attracted to New Zealand and helped to introduce the British block system of nursing education. Nursing textbooks and British journals had an influence in strengthening the British system.[10]

Most nurses in New Zealand are prepared in Hospital Board Schools of Nursing, which are service based and hospital oriented. As many as 139 basic nursing programs leading to registration are offered by these schools. The male nurse course is the same as the general nurse course but has less emphasis on obstetrical nursing. The psychopaedic course prepared nurses to work with mentally retarded children, and the community nurse course is equivalent to the practical nurse course in the United States.[9]

The existence of separate courses at the basic level stems from the historically separate administration of general and specialized hospitals. In 1972 responsibility for the maintenance of psychopaedic, psychiatric, and midwifery services was transferred from the Department of Health to Hospital Boards. Separate administration has led to the development of different registration requirements, different curricula, and a different career and salary structure.[9]

Since the general nursing course does not offer enough experience in maternity nursing, the majority of registered nurses take the six-month postbasic course, which qualifies them as maternity nurses. A full twelve-month midwifery course at the postgraduate level came into being in 1930.

In addition, the Royal New Zealand Society for the Health of Women and Children (Plunket Society), offered a four-month course to registered nurses interested in working in infant welfare and mothercraft agencies.[2,5]

Also, in 1928 a six-month postgraduate course in hospital and training school administration and public health nursing was available to nurses interested in higher education. This course was run by the Department of Health with the cooperation of Victoria University, the Wellington Hospital public health services, and other social services in the country.[1,2]

Students in Hospital Schools of Nursing in New Zealand are employees of the Hospital Boards. They work 8-hour shifts in a 40-hour work week. In the three-year general course, students receive a three-month introductory course during which they enjoy full student status. For the remainder of the three years the block system is adopted, during which students may have approximately a hundred study days, depending on the method adopted by the school. The Nursing Council of New Zealand prescribes the minimum number of theoretical hours and the content of the courses offered at the schools. Clinical experience also is planned and prescribed by the council and requires one month of training in a community health center and one to three months in a psychiatric hospital. Rostering students for service leaves little chance of correlating theory with practice and thus results in the inevitable subordination of education to service.[9]

The nursing education system in New Zealand does not produce the kind of nurse that the country needs. The Division of Nursing, Department of Health, New Zealand Registered Nurses' Association, and New Zealand Student Nurses' Association have done their best to point out the weaknesses of such a system. In addition, the reports of the World Health Organization Expert Committee on Nursing and the Review of Hospitals and Related Services have contributed to an increase in government interest in nursing education and the need for change. The main goal behind the movement for change is the transfer of the education of nursing from the Department of Health to the Department of Education. This places nursing education in the general education system and replaces the separate three-year programs with a single comprehensive basic course.[9]

Since Hospital Boards form an important political force in the country, they managed to provide an obstacle to the removal of nursing schools from their realm of authority. They believe that the maintenance of such schools in a hospital setting ensures a continuous supply of trained nurses. This belief was supported by the government, which views the work force that students represent in the hospital system as an important asset.[9]

CHANGE IN NURSING EDUCATION

Basic courses in nursing education are in transition. The technical institute programs embody the major themes of the desired change that has been voiced throughout the past few years. Such a program gives complete student status to the participant, is not dominated by demands from hospital service, and offers an equal share of theory and practice. Furthermore, such a program integrates family and community health in its course structure, focusing more on the community than on the hospital. All these programs are presently offered outside the hospital boundaries, that is, within the Department of Education.[11]

However, the School of Advanced Nursing Studies, formerly known as the postgraduate school, is still under the Department of Health. The nine-month course covers subjects in the management of nursing service, nursing education, and public health nursing. Within the Department of Health two new programs have emerged lately: a regional course for qualified nurses in community health, offered at four technical institutes, and a course for nurse tutors, offered at Wellington and Hamilton Teachers' Colleges.[11]

Postbasic courses at the Universities of Victoria and Massey are expanding in terms of programs and students. The Victoria University offers courses in nursing studies to be included in the Bachelor of Arts program. Massey University offers a diploma program in addition to the nursing studies course. The course on nursing studies at Massey is presently a part of the postgraduate area of study in nursing, offering both the Bachelor of Arts (Honours) and the master's degrees. Postbasic nursing programs continue to be offered at Massey University providing refresher courses, mainly in clinical and technical subjects, to nurses throughout New Zealand.[1,11] (See Table 2.)

The basic nursing programs at the Nelson and Wellington Polytechnics and the Christchurch and Auckland Technical Institutes are progressing well. The Department of Education Research and Planning Unit is responsible for the ongoing evaluation of these programs. Graduate nurses of the technical institutes are registered as comprehensive nurses and are employed in a variety of settings in the health services centers of the country. Private hospitals are phasing out their hospital-based schools of nursing. However, the country is left with twenty-seven hospital schools that offer three-year general/male nursing courses, three-year psychiatric nursing courses, three-year psychopaedic nursing courses, eighteen-month community nurse courses, six-month maternity nursing courses, and six-month midwifery courses. Much attention has been given lately to assisting these schools to improve the education and training of student nurses.[7]

HEALTH SERVICES

Two alternatives are available for operation of the health care delivery system in New Zealand: One is known as the medical model and the other as the health model. The difference between the two concepts, medical and

TABLE 2
Levels of nursing education in New Zealand

Level	Type of course	Length of course	Registration
Basic	General nurse	3 years	RGN
	Male nurse	3 years	R Male N
	Psychiatric nurse	3 years	RPN
	Psychopaedic nurse	3 years	R Psychopaedic nurse
	Community nurse	18 months	RCN
	Comprehensive course in nursing	3 years	RN
Postbasic	Midwifery	6 months	RM
	Management of nursing service	9 months	
	Nursing education	9 months	
	Public health	9 months	
Graduate	Nursing studies at Victoria and Massey Universities	Varies	B.A. degree
Postgraduate	Nursing studies at Massey University	Varies	Honours and master's degrees

health, is related to the location of authority regarding decisions in the health field. If the medical model is adopted, decisions on health matters are concerned with medical and curative matters. In such a case nurses and other paramedical professionals apply the medical decisions, and their role is mainly the intelligent execution of the required tasks. Decisions of a medical type can be made by a nurse only in the absence of a physician, which means that the nurse will then have acted outside his or her legitimate role.[4,6,11]

The health model takes a different base for authority by involving patients, physicians, nurses, and other paramedical personnel in the decision-making process. In this model the emphasis is on the synthesis of all decisions around and with the patient. The responsibility and accountability of each health professional are considered in terms of that person's area of expertise.[4]

Responsibility for the nation's health lies in the hands of central and local government, private medical practitioners, paramedical workers, charitable and religious organizations, and private citizens. The central government contributes to the country's health services by providing encouragement, incentives, and financial assistance. The Department of Health is responsible for the organization and control of nursing services in general, which include the supervision of hospitals, homes for the aged, and public health agencies. A great deal of delegation has been moved to Hospital Boards, where the chief nursing officer is directly responsible to the chief medical officer in the day-to-day execution of health services.[3]

Under the Social Security Act, medical practitioners give prenatal, neonatal, and postnatal care. Free antenatal clinics are established in maternity hospitals and wards as well as general hospitals throughout the country. Antenatal classes prepare parents for the arrival of their babies. In New Zealand most of the confinements take place in maternity hospitals or in maternity units of public hospitals. Maternal and child health services are the responsibility of the Department of Health, Hospital Boards, medical and nursing professions, and the Royal New Zealand Society for the Health of Women and Children (Plunket Society). In addition, the Department of Health provides a preventive child health service, physicians performing the initial examination of infants and public health nurses undertaking supervision and follow-up.[3]

Although the team approach to the provision of primary health services has been slow to develop in New Zealand, the role of the nurse in primary health care is becoming better defined. In 1970 the first subsidized practice nurse scheme was introduced for rural physicians, resulting in increased utilization of practice nurses. A second subsidized scheme was introduced in 1974 for physicians working in rural and urban areas, producing an increase in the employment of practice nurses in urban centers. The wide range of nursing skills available in general practice, according to a survey done in 1975, has contributed greatly to the improvement in the quality of health care provided. It was found that nurses eased the work load of physicians, enabling the latter to care for a larger number of patients. Many medical and technical procedures, traditionally done by physicians, are being delegated to nurses. Undoubtedly this aspect of nursing care will increase, and extensive use of practice nurses and other members of the health team will become more acceptable to the population. A not uncommon experience is for a patient to ask to be seen by a nurse rather than by a physician.[7]

REFERENCES

1. Boyd, E.: Postbasic nursing education in New Zealand, International Nursing Review **17**(1):43-52, 1970.
2. Bridges, E. R.: Nursing in New Zealand, American Journal of Nursing **39:**1205-1212, 1939.
3. Health and hospitals, New Zealand Official Yearbook **5:**124-140, 1974.
4. Mordacq, C.: Constraints and opportunities in a nursing career, International Nursing Review **20:**112-113, July-Aug., 1973.
5. Nursing in New Zealand, American Journal of Nursing **47:**216-217, 1947.
6. Penman, H. G.: Health service reorganization, New Zealand Medical Journal **82**(543):22-23, 1975.

7. Report of the Department of Health: The public health, Wellington, 1976, New Zealand Department of Health.
8. Report of the Nursing Council of New Zealand: The nursing council of New Zealand, Wellington, 1976, Nursing Council of New Zealand.
9. Shadbolt, Y. T.: Nursing education in New Zealand, The New Zealand Nursing Journal **68**(1):19-22, 1975.
10. Stewart, I., and Austin, A.: A history of nursing, New York, 1962, G. P. Putnam's Sons.
11. Thomson, M.: Change in nursing education, The New Zealand Nursing Journal **68**(12):22-23, 1975.

LOOKING AHEAD

NURSING PRACTICE

Over the past few years, many experiments on the availability, quality, and scope of health care have taken place. Such experiments dealt with the expanded role of professionals in nursing and the different ways in which paraprofessionals could be utilized. The movement toward expanding the role of the nurse evolved recently, prompted by different social forces such as consumer demands for higher quality care and better distribution of health care facilities. The nursing profession also has witnessed an increased number of nurses seeking advanced nursing education as clinical specialists and nurse practitioners. This new movement led nurses to rebel against the health system and, as a result, adopt new titles such as family nurse practitioners, pediatric nurse practitioners, geriatric nurse practitioners, primary nurses, direct care nurses, rural health practitioners, adult health practitioners, medical nurse practitioners, and psychiatric nurse practitioners.[1]

The shift in perspective from medical care to health care is a recent trend. The health care concept places more emphasis on prevention and health maintenance than did the medical care concept, which emphasized mainly treatment of the sick. Nurses are gaining recognition throughout the world as providers of primary health care. In the United States the question about direct reimbursement for nonphysician providers has been considered by Congress. The variety of approaches for reimbursement include (1) nonprofit group practices of nurses, (2) health maintenance organizations, (3) rural and urban nurse clinics, and (4) home health nursing services. Nurses in the United States believe that they have the right to be recognized as providers of care, thus making them eligible for direct reimbursement just as are dentists, optometrists, physicians, podiatrists, and psychologists.[4]

The role of nurse practitioner requires more than the gaining of new skills in medicine and nursing; it requires a complete reorientation of the nurse to a totally new career that requires greater independence and responsibility. The transition period will result in the modification of social and professional norms, attitudes, and values as an outcome of the newly perceived role. These changes will be accompanied by a great deal of physical, social, and psychological stress as nurses move from their traditional role to one that emphasizes nursing assessment and decision making. Additional stresses include the development of a viable relationship with medical co-workers, who are at times misinformed about the nurse practitioners' functions and who therefore feel threatened by this new type of health care worker.[1]

To reach a mutual understanding of the role and functions of a nurse practitioner, the American Medical Association and the American Nurses' Association have held a series of joint conferences. The National Joint Practice Commission was an outgrowth of these efforts. The commission, which includes eight physicians and eight nurses, has published a book, *Together—a Casebook of Joint Practice in Primary Care,* which considers innovations in joint practice in the health care field.[2] In addition to serving on the commission, physicians have served on committees to develop guidelines for nurse practitioner programs. Physicians have also assisted in writing test items for the certification examinations for pediatric nurse practitioners and family and adult nurse practitioners.[1]

NURSING EDUCATION

The knowledge explosion coupled with rapidly growing technology will affect the way nursing will be taught in the future. Maximizing education for individuals will be the goal of the coming century. To be prepared for the more demanding future, nurses throughout the world will need to be aware of nursing and medical trends and developments. Faced with such massive social concerns—not only the knowledge explosion but the energy crisis, resource depletion, world hunger, and overpopulation—many countries are turning to the computer for assistance. In Japan, for example, the individual model on which society is built is being replaced by the information model. This newly planned society is known as the "information society." In such a society the computer will undoubtedly play an important role in manipulating and storing the vast amount of data available in a far more orderly fashion than humans could do by conventional methods.[5]

The classical role of the teacher as the primary transmitter of knowledge is undoubtedly disappearing. New and innovative teaching methods such as programmed instruction, learning modules, computer-based or computer-managed instruction, and various other strategies classified as individualized instruction are becoming increasingly popular. As a result, the teacher will become more of a facilitator of learning, allowing technology to participate in the teaching/learning process. In the future the use of the computer will be widespread in some parts of the world, helping the teacher to manage the increasingly complex educational environment. Such an effort will include instruction, evaluation, identification of problems, data gathering, data manipulation for research, and continuing education. Some countries have already utilized the computer in some of these areas, whereas others are still experimenting.

The accelerated rate of change and its far-reaching implications for all institutions in society has always had its effect on the nursing profession. Nurses believe that change is fundamental to the survival of the profession. A general agreement among nursing educators in the world is that reliable and relevant knowledge must be put to good use to meet human needs. As a result, nursing faculty are continuously engaged in improving their curricula by making changes to affect the quality of the educational experiences that students receive. Such a trend is envisioned as being vital to the profession only if new developments in nursing curricula are based on a foundation of validated knowledge. Nursing educators, like other educators, should look critically at innovations before adopting major curricular changes, especially at this time when the profession is moving into full professional status.

WORLD HEALTH AND NURSING

After an examination of the various methods used by countries throughout the world in providing health care, a general conclusion can be drawn that in both developed and developing countries the health care delivery system does not meet the needs of the whole population. To remedy this, the World Health Organization introduced the primary health care concept in 1975. Although such an approach differs from one country to another, the following general principles form a baseline:

1. Primary health care is shaped around the life patterns of the population and hence meets the community's needs.
2. Primary health care constitutes an integral part of the national health system.
3. Primary health care forms a part of the activities involved in community development.
4. Local communities are actively involved in the formulation and implementation of health care activities.
5. Health care provided places a reliance on available resources in the community and falls within the financial limitations of the country.
6. Primary health care integrates the concepts of prevention, promotion, cure, and rehabilitation in its effort to serve the individual, family, and community.
7. Health services are provided at the practical level by personnel trained to perform these activities.[3]

In adopting these baseline principles to provide primary health care at the community level throughout the world, changes in the curricula and training of physicians, nurses, and midwives should be introduced. This will enable these health professionals to provide the health care services that the community needs. In addition, changes in training programs of other health personnel, professional and paraprofessional, will provide the team orientation concept, helping the primary health workers become an integral part of the communities they serve.

The provision of primary health care to every segment of the population is today's most crucial health problem. The training of members of the community as primary health workers offers a realistic approach in providing health care services to millions of people. The community health nurse will essentially assume more responsibilities in the training of the primary health workers and in serving as a link between them and the rest of the health care system.

To meet the growing needs for health care, nurses of the future will be more community oriented. More community nursing services will be developed to provide primary health coverage for every segment of the population. As a result, nursing manpower will constitute a major part in the health manpower scheme, creating a challenge for nurses and placing more responsibility on them in the health care delivery system.

ETHICAL CONCEPTS IN NURSING

Change is considered to be constant in today's society, which is always in a transient stage. Many honored institutions in society, such as the family and church, have taken on different appearances. Along with this movement, many ethical concepts in nursing have changed, to be outgrown by the several directions that the profession is presently taking. Ethical codes are drawn from real-life situations, making use of present and past experiences to look for the future.

Ethical concepts in the future might move from the curative-preventive dichotomy to focus on the adaptation of the individual to social change. Death will be looked at by nurses as an integral part of the life process, and they will recognize the right of individuals to determine how they want to end their lives. In the future the nurse will be called on to develop innovative standards to meet the changing needs of society. Competence through education and practice will be the future yardstick. Togetherness rather than separation of roles is the envisioned role that health workers might take to provide patient care. Each member of the health team will contribute to the provision of health care in a holistic approach, according to that person's area of specialization. Community involvement and consumer control of health services will be the trend. Such a system will help to bridge the gap between the physician or other health worker and the patient. In addition, outreach services will be available in an attempt to provide health services for the aged, the handicapped, the battered child, and the lay person in every nation.

These few thoughts on the future of nursing emphasize personal responsibility for nursing practice, the commitment of nurses to the welfare of society, and their sense of responsibility to speak up when an issue is at stake. Nursing has witnessed great change, but the future is more promising and presents a challenge to the nurses of the world.

REFERENCES

1. Apostoles, E.: Role expansion in a psychiatric setting, Nurse Practitioner **2:**22-25, 1976.
2. Berton, R., editor: Together—a casebook of joint practice in primary care, Chicago, 1977, The National Joint Practice Commission.
3. Hentsch, Y.: Community and world health, International Nursing Review **23:** 103-106, July-Aug., 1976.
4. Jennings, C.: Third party reimbursement and the nurse practitioner, Nurse Practitioner **2:**11-13, 1977.
5. Meadows, L.: Nursing education in crisis, a computer alternative, Journal of Nursing Education **16:**13-21, 1977.

Appendix

Summary of nursing from ancient to modern times

Florence Nightingale's creation of St. Thomas's Hospital School of Nursing in 1860 was the beginning of what is now known as "modern nursing"—modern meaning the progress of nursing in the context of its marked phase of development and period of time. The contribution of Florence Nightingale was the founding of a profession based on scientific innovation and medical knowledge. Thus an independent, self-supporting profession for women of education, culture, and social standing was founded on a secular, humanitarian, and strictly feminist basis.

General events and movements, shared by the different countries mentioned in this book, have had their impact on the development of the profession. The increasing number of wars in recent centuries has led to increased participation of nurses in military service. In addition, liberal, democratic, social, and labor movements have placed a value on the health of the individual, family, and community, broadening the role of the nurse in this area. Colonial powers have also contributed to the establishment of nursing systems in some Asian and African countries. The Russian and Chinese revolutions have introduced ideologies that influenced the direction of nursing in some parts of the world.

Although modern nursing services were generally nonsectarian, religious orders that played an important role in establishing nursing schools through their mission work around the world have continued to administer and support hospitals and schools of nursing until the present. Nurse missionaries were sent to foreign countries, carrying with them modern nursing systems of training. During the same period, social and civil agencies were developing—a movement that helped to introduce the Nightingale

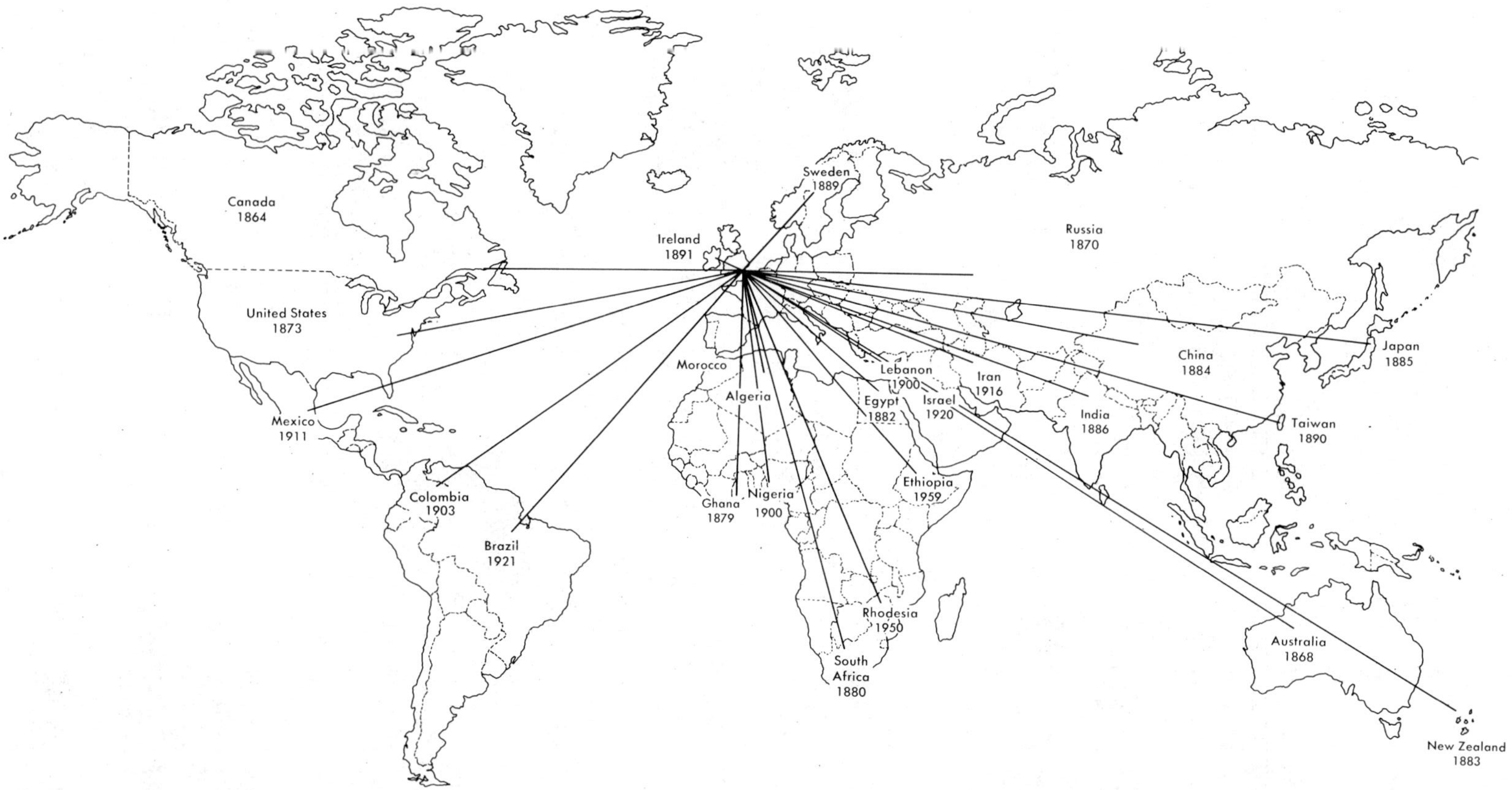

Canada 1864
United States 1873
Mexico 1911
Colombia 1903
Brazil 1921
Ireland 1891
Sweden 1889
Russia 1870
Morocco
Algeria
Ghana 1879
Nigeria 1900
Egypt 1882
Lebanon 1900
Israel 1920
Iran 1916
Ethiopia 1959
Rhodesia 1950
South Africa 1880
India 1886
China 1884
Japan 1885
Taiwan 1890
Australia 1868
New Zealand 1883

FIG. 14

Development of modern nursing.

nursing reforms to the already existing nursing systems of the countries. Fig. 14 shows the influence of the Nightingale system on the development of modern nursing practices in many countries.

The Red Cross movement has also had an influence on the profession. Red Cross, founded in 1864, concentrated on training nurses to serve in wars and natural disasters. However, in times of peace, nurses were trained for private duty, visiting nursing, and hospital service. Red Cross schools of nursing throughout the world have attracted women from the upper middle and even higher social classes, thus raising the standards of the profession.

Noteworthy is the contribution of the World Health Organization to the development of nursing in several countries. This international organization through its different offices has helped in organizing programs and, in some places, creating training centers for the preparation of nurses in various specialties. The World Health Organization also made material contributions to some developing countries and some of these nations are still dependent on this assistance.

Although primitive nursing was done mostly by the servant class of society in most countries, many leaders of the profession have emerged from cultured homes to establish the roots of the modern nursing system. The development of nursing as a profession seems to have gone hand in hand with the international women's movement. The better educational opportunities for girls, society's acceptance of women seeking careers, and the availability of nursing schools as an academic route have had an impact on attracting young women of education and culture into the profession.

The dominant trend among all countries included in this book has been toward the recognition of nursing as a profession, distinct from other health professions. In some countries nursing is an independent, self-supporting profession, whereas in others it is still under medical control. The professional development of nursing throughout the world has been accompanied by the establishment of national associations, leading to membership in the international nursing organization. In addition, nursing legislation for the control of nursing practice and education through registration of nurses and accreditation of nursing schools was another movement shared by nurses of the world. Table 3 shows how nursing associations have affected nursing registration and membership in the International Council of Nurses in most countries of the world, with the exception of Nigeria, New Zealand, and South Africa.

The education of nurses, professional and nonprofessional, basic and advanced, has included similar trends and movements. Schools of nursing in most countries are recognized as separate institutions independent from the hospital system. Nursing education at the basic level is considered to be a branch of professional work in some countries, whereas in others it is

TABLE 3

Nursing registration and organization

Country	Nursing associations	Nursing registration	ICN membership
Australia	1899	1927	1937
Brazil	1925	1931	1929
Canada	1899	1922	1909
China	1909	1937	1922
Egypt			1961
England	1888	1889	1900
Ethiopia			1957
France	1923	1922	1925
Germany	1903	1905	1904
Ghana	1946	1946	1961
Greece	1923	1948	1929
Holland	1892	1921	1928
India	1905	1923	1912
Ireland	1925	1950	1947
Israel	1953		1953
Italy	1920	1954	1946
Japan	1925	1948	1925
Lebanon		1932	1969
Mexico	1947		1961
New Zealand	1908	1901	1912
Nigeria	1946	1910	1961
Rhodesia			1949
Russia	1938	1935	
South Africa	1914	1891	1922
Sweden	1910	1920	1929
Taiwan			1961
United States of America	1893	1903-1923	1900
Yugoslavia	1926	1931	1929

still at the technical level. Many countries have placed nursing education among other programs that are offered in higher educational institutions. The establishment of university nursing programs at basic and graduate levels is a worldwide trend. In some countries university nursing education is the most common movement, whereas in others this constitutes a future goal. Table 4 lists the levels of educational practices in the countries included in this book.

Fields of nursing service have multiplied rapidly during recent decades. At the present time emphasis is on the concepts of prevention and positive health. With the expanded role of the nurse, conditions of practice have also improved, giving nurses more responsibility in the health care delivery system. Nursing personnel throughout the world are prepared at different

Text continued on p. 219.

TABLE 4
Levels of nursing education in the world

Country	Basic	Postbasic	Graduate	Auxiliary
Algeria	Paramedical centers General nursing, 2 years Midwifery, 2 years			Nurses' aides, 11 months
Australia	Hospital-based schools General nursing, 3 years Colleges of advanced nursing education Diploma nursing, 3 years	Nursing education Nursing administration Nursing management		Auxiliary nurses
Brazil	University schools Professional nursing, 4 years Technical schools Diploma nursing, 3 years	Public health nursing Nursing education Nursing administration	Master's degree Nursing education Nursing administration	Practical nurses, 1½ years
Canada	University schools Professional nursing, 4 years Schools of nursing Diploma nursing, 2 years	Public health nursing	Nurse-midwifery Master's degree Nurse practitioner Nursing research	Nurses' aides Assistant nurses, 1 year
China	Barefoot doctor college Barefoot doctor, 2 years Schools of nursing General nursing, 2 years			Barefoot doctors, 4 months
Colombia	University schools Professional nursing or licentiate in nursing science, 4 years Schools of nursing General nursing, 3 years		Master's degree Maternal-child nursing Psychiatric nursing Medical and surgical nursing	Practical nurses, 1½ years Nurses' aides, 3 months
Cuba	Schools of nursing Diploma nursing, 3½ years	Obstetrical nursing Pediatric nursing Adult nursing Nursing administration Teaching		Promotors of health, 3 months

Continued.

TABLE 4
Levels of nursing education in the world—cont'd

Country	Basic	Postbasic	Graduate	Auxiliary
Egypt	University schools Professional nursing, 5 years Schools of nursing Diploma nursing, 3 years		Master's degree Preventive health and nursing	
England	Hospital-based schools General nursing, 3 years University schools Professional nursing, 4 years	Midwifery Health visiting District nursing Administration Teaching	Clinical practitioners Research	Assistant nurses, 2 years Practical nurses Nurses' aides Home helpers
Ethiopia	Schools of nursing Diploma nursing, 3½ to 4 years			
France	Schools of nursing General nursing, 3 years Psychiatric nursing, 2 years Assistante sociale, 3½ years Midwifery schools Midwives, 3 years	Head nursing Nursing service administration Nursing school administration Public health nursing		
Germany	University schools Professional nursing, 4 years Hospital-based schools Diploma nursing, 3 years	Clinical specialist	Public health nursing Nursing education	Assistant nurses, 1 year Nurses' aides, 1 year
Ghana	Schools of nursing Diploma nursing, 3 years Nurse-midwifery schools Nurse-midwives, 3 years	Nursing education Nursing administration Public health nursing		Nursing assistants Community health nurses
Greece	Schools of nursing General nursing, 3 years Schools of midwifery Midwifery, 3 years	Public health nursing		Practical nurses, 1 year Nurses' aides

	Diploma nursing, 3 years Higher education nursing schools Professional nursing, 4 years			
India	Schools of nursing Diploma nursing, 3 years University schools Professional nursing, 4 years	Nursing administration Nursing education Pediatric nursing Midwifery Public health nursing	Master's degree Clinical specialist Education Administration International health	Nurse-midwives, 2 years Health visitors, 2½ years
Iran	Schools of nursing Diploma nursing, 3 years University schools Professional nursing, 4 years	Midwifery		Practical nurses, 2 years Public health nurses, 2 years
Ireland	Hospital-based schools General nursing, 3 years Psychiatric nursing, 3 years Pediatric nursing, 3 years Mentally handicapped nursing, 3 years	Nurse tutors Clinical specialists		
Israel	Hospital-based schools Diploma nursing, 3 years University schools Professional nursing, 4 years	Public health nursing Midwifery Operating-room techniques Mental health nursing		Practical nurses, 1½ years Nurses' aides
Italy	Hospital-based schools General nursing, 2 years Children's nursing, 2 years Midwifery, 3 years	Head nursing Public health nursing Nursing education		Practical nurses, 1 year
Japan	Schools of nursing Diploma nursing, 3 years Schools for assistant nurses Diploma nursing, 3 years University schools Professional nursing, 4 years	Public health nursing Midwifery Nurse tutors Nursing administration		Assistant nurses, 2 years

Continued.

TABLE 4
Levels of nursing education in the world—cont'd

Country	Basic	Postbasic	Graduate	Auxiliary
Lebanon	University schools Professional nursing, 4 years Schools of nursing Diploma nursing, 3 years Psychiatric nursing, 3 years Technical schools Technical baccalaureate Part I nursing, 2 years Technical baccalaureate Part II nursing, 4 years	Public health nursing Nursing education Nursing administration Clinical specialist Midwifery	Master's degree Public health nursing Midwifery	Practical nurses' 6 to 12 months Nurses' aides
Mexico	University schools Professional nursing, 4 years Schools of nursing General nursing, 3 years	Public health nursing		
Morocco	Schools of nursing Diploma nursing, 2 years Psychiatric nursing, 2 years Obstetrical nursing, 2 years	Nursing education Nursing administration Obstetrical nursing		Auxiliary nurses, 19 months
New Zealand	Hospital-based schools General nursing, 3 years Psychiatric nursing, 3 years Psychopaedic nursing, 3 years Community nursing, 1½ years Schools of nursing Comprehensive nursing, 3 years University programs Nursing studies	Nursing service management Nursing education Public health Midwifery Clinical specialization		

	Diploma nursing, 3½ years
	  Midwifery, 1 year
	  Community health nursing, 3 years
	University schools
	  Professional nursing, 3 years
		Public health nursing
		Community health nursing
				wives

Rhodesia	Schools of nursing Diploma nursing, 3 years	Midwifery Psychiatric nursing Advanced clinical nursing		

Russia	Schools of nursing
	  Basic nursing
	    Sestras, 3 years
	    Fledshers, 3½ years
		Midwifery
		Public health nursing
		Pediatric nursing
		Head nursing
		Anesthesiology
		Surgical nursing
		Physical therapy
		Psychiatry
			Medical degree	Nurses' aides
				Orderlies

South Africa	Nursing colleges
	  Basic nursing, 3½ years
	University schools
	  Professional nursing, 4½ years
	Bantu colleges
	  Basic nursing, 3½ years
	Midwifery schools
	  Midwifery, 1½ years
		Nursing administration
		Clinical specialization
		Midwifery
		Nursing education
		Public health nursing
		Occupational health nursing
			Master's degree
			  Nursing education
			  Nursing administration
			  Clinical nursing
			Doctoral degree research
				Nurses' aides

Sweden	Schools of nursing General nursing, 2½ years	Pediatric nursing Operating-room techniques Midwifery Nursing education Nursing administration Clinical nursing		Practical nurses, 32 weeks Nurses' aides, 7 weeks

Continued.

TABLE 4
Levels of nursing education in the world—cont'd

Country	Basic	Postbasic	Graduate	Auxiliary
Taiwan	Vocational schools Diploma nursing, 3 years University schools Professional nursing, 4 years Midwifery, 4 years Nursing colleges Professional nursing, 3 years Midwifery, 3 years Technical colleges Clinical practitioners, 5 years	Public health nursing Midwifery		
United States of America	University schools Professional nursing, 4 years Community colleges Technical nursing, 2 years Schools of nursing Diploma nursing, 3 years	Nurse clinician Nurse practitioner	Master's degree Clinical specialization Public health nursing Nurse-midwifery Nursing education Nursing administration Nurse practitioner Doctoral degree Nursing science Nursing research Nursing education	Practical nurses, 1 year Nurses' aides
Yugoslavia	Advanced schools of nursing Professional nursing, 3 years Middle medical schools Diploma nursing, 4 years Midwifery, 4 years Pediatric nursing, 4 years	Teaching Head nursing Midwifery Operating-room techniques Nurse dietetics Public health nursing		Assistant nurses, 2 years

TABLE 5
Primary health care workers

Country	Title	Program started	Level of education
Australia	Bush nurses	1909	Basic
Canada	Nurse practitioners	1972	Graduate
China	Barefoot doctors	1949	Basic and auxiliary
England	Nurse practitioners or health visitors	1948	Basic and postbasic
Holland	Family nurse practitioners and pediatric nurse practitioners	1970	Basic and postbasic
Iran	Primary health workers		Auxiliary
Israel	Kibbutz nurses	1948	Basic
Nigeria	Community health nurses and child health nurses	1950	Postbasic
Rhodesia	Advanced clinical nurses		Postbasic
Russia	*Fledshers*	1917	Basic
Sweden	Clinical specialists		Postbasic
United States of America	Nurse practitioners	1971	Basic and graduate

levels to supplement the physician in providing primary health care. These primary health workers are taking the role belonging to the family doctor in the past. Table 5 shows the various titles these health workers have used and compares their level of educational preparation in certain countries.

Nursing conditions, including regulation of supply and demand, conditions of work, hours, salaries, and pensions, have improved in most countries. This is partly because of increased government involvement and the interest of professional and nursing organizations in matters that concern the future development of the profession. In addition, nursing journals and other communication channels have helped nurses to interpret nursing to the public and have kept the profession abreast with new developments. Nursing surveys, studies, and research conducted in some countries have improved the quality of nursing care and contributed to the advancement of the profession at the international level.

Nurses working across national boundaries have had a significant share in the development of their profession. They have shown the world that they could rise above intolerance and inhumanity, fighting abuses but keeping their fraternal spirits and international aims. Broadening their knowledge about nursing practices in other countries ensures better cooperation and friendship among nurses of the world. This constitutes the best hope for nurses of the future and for a profession that is dedicated to the service of humanity and world peace.

INDEX